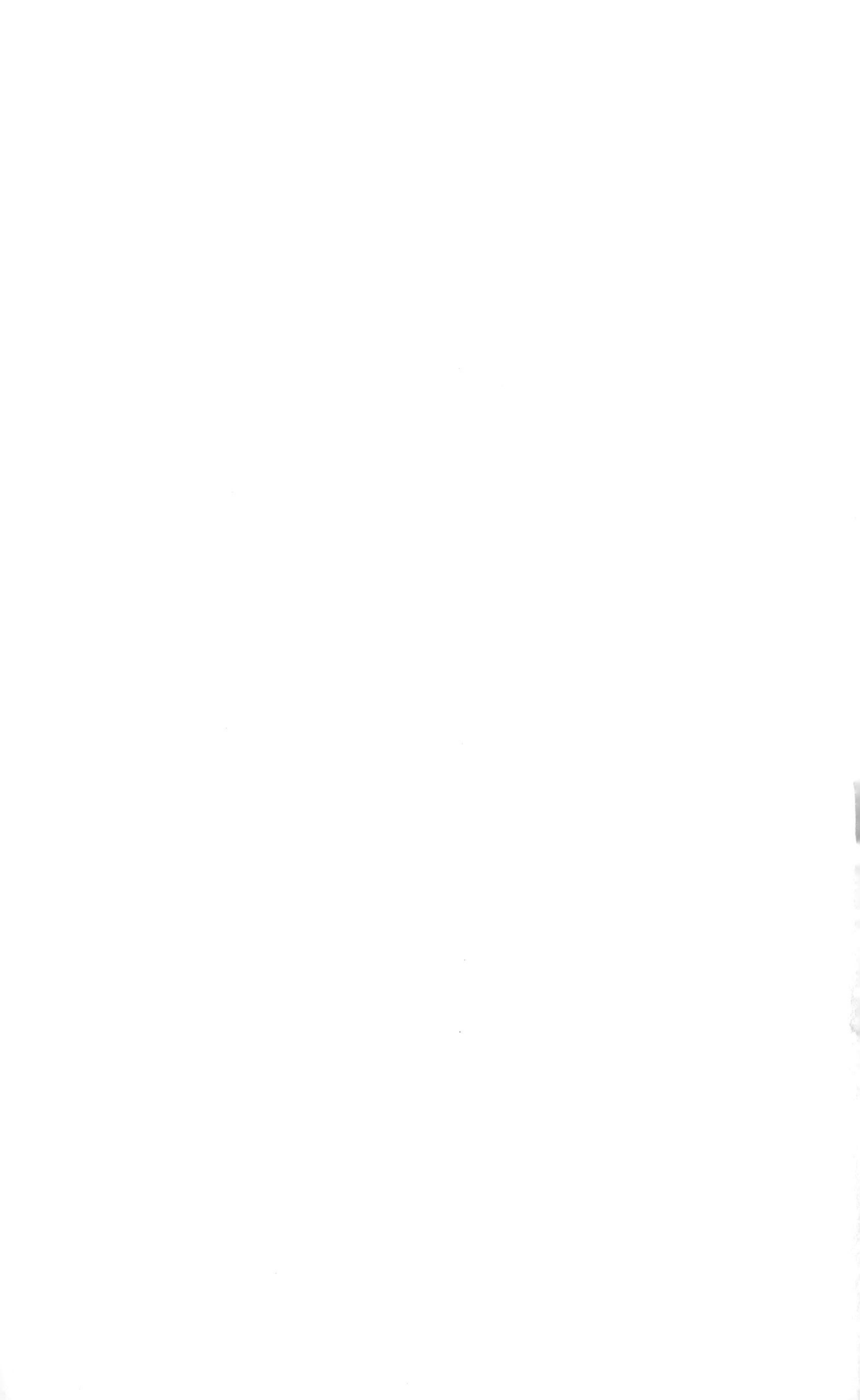

12 DAY POWER *Detox*

Revive, Restore and Rejuvenate Your Spirit, Soul and Body!

12 Day Power Detox

Revive, Restore and Rejuvenate your spirit, soul and body!

© 2019 Adewunmi Ashaye & It's Time Fitness LLC
All Rights Reserved

Cover & Design Layout by CHiCPEA Studios

Published by: It's Time Fitness LLC

ISBNs
13: 978-1-7336880-0-0 (pb)
13: 978-1-7336880-1-7 (hc)
13: 978-1-7336880-2-4 (eb)

DEDICATION

This book is dedicated to God, the Source of this life-changing book; my family and friends for their support and encouragement; my ever-growing fitness community for believing in the transformational power of the 12 Day Power Detox; and finally, to everyone who worked behind the scene to make this book a reality. I love and appreciate you all.

12 DAY POWER DETOX

Revive, Restore and Rejuvenate your spirit, soul and body!

- ➤ Includes meal and activity plan, grocery list and delicious smoothie recipes.
- ➤ Release unwanted weight, up to fifteen pounds.
- ➤ Revive your body with essential living foods while eliminating harmful toxins.
- ➤ Restore by replenishing your body with nutrients that can easily be absorbed.
- ➤ Retrain your stomach to love nature's best foods and reject counterfeits.
- ➤ Regain energy with powerful superfoods.
- ➤ Rejuvenate your soul and spirit by detoxing negative emotions with the included 12 Day Power Detox Devotional.

CONTENTS

WAIVER 7

INTRODUCTION 8

    THE BIRTH OF THE POWER DETOX PROGRAM 9

CHAPTER 1 – THE ANATOMY OF A GREEN SMOOTHIE

    BENEFITS OF GREEN SMOOTHIES DETOX 14

    WHAT'S IN YOUR SMOOTHIE CUP? 16

    HOW TO MAKE A DETOX SMOOTHIE 16

CHAPTER 2 – PREPARING FOR THE DETOX PROGRAM

    IMPORTANT NOTES 20

    PREP WEEK 22

    GROCERY LIST 23

    FOODS TO AVOID ON THE DETOX PROGRAM...........................24

    FREQUENTLY ASKED QUESTIONS (F.A.Q.) 25

CHAPTER 3 – THE PROGRAM

    SMOOTHIE RECIPES 32

        SMOOTHIE MEAL PORTIONS 32

        WEEK 1 SMOOTHIE RECIPES 32

        WEEK 2 SMOOTHIE RECIPES 34

        WEEK 1 MEAL AND ACTIVITY PLAN (M.A.P.) 36

        WEEK 2 MEAL AND ACTIVITY PLAN (M.A.P.) 37

    TROPICAL SMOOTHIE RECIPES 38

        PREP WEEK 38

        GROCERY LIST 39

        WEEK 1 SMOOTHIE RECIPES 40

        WEEK 2 SMOOTHIE RECIPES 42

WEEK 1 MEAL AND ACTIVITY PLAN (M.A.P.) 44

WEEK 2 MEAL AND ACTIVITY PLAN (M.A.P.) 45

SNACKS..46

SPICE UP YOUR SMOOTHIE 46

CHAPTER 4 – AFTER THE PROGRAM

AFTER THE 12 DAY POWER DETOX PROGRAM 52

SAMPLE HEALTHY EATING RECIPES 52

CHAPTER 5 – 12 DAY POWER DETOX DEVOTIONAL

INTRODUCTION 56

THE EMOTIONAL DETOX PROCESS 57

DAY 1: CREATE IN ME A CLEAN HEART 62

DAY 2: LET GO, LET GOD - UNFORGIVENESS 65

DAY 3: LET IT GO - UNFORGIVENESS 69

DAY 4: DEALING WITH OVERWHELMING FEELINGS............73

DAY 5: DEALING WITH JOY KILLERS 79

DAY 6: DEALING WITH UNFULFILLED EXPECTATIONS 85

DAY 7: DEALING WITH ACCUSATIONS 91

DAY 8: DEALING WITH DISCONTENTMENT 96

DAY 9: DEALING WITH SELF IDOLATRY..............................102

DAY 10: DEALING WITH ADDICTIONS AND CRAVINGS 108

DAY 11: POWER OF SPOKEN WORDS 116

DAY 12: DEALING WITH REJECTION 124

CHAPTER 6 – SUCCESS STORIES & TESTIMONIALS

SUCCESS STORIES 134

TESTIMONIALS 148

BECOME A 12 DAY POWER DETOX AMBASSADOR 149

ABOUT THE AUTHOR 151

WAIVER

By participating in 12 Day Power Detox Program, you are agreeing to our terms and conditions at **www.itstimefitnessaz.com/terms**.

Please consult with your physician before beginning this or any diet program.

As with any health or fitness program, if at any point, you begin to feel faint, dizzy, or have physical discomfort, you should stop immediately and consult a physician.

INTRODUCTION

The 12 Day Power Detox Program is an intensive 12-day nutrition and wellness program created by Divine inspiration—JUST FOR YOU!

The *nutrition* part of the program comprises of a 12-day green smoothie meal plan which will help you detox harmful toxins from your body. The *wellness* part comprises a 12-day Devotional which will help you detox negative emotions from your soul while embracing positive emotions. This brings a unique and holistic approach to our program.

This is not a weight loss program, but participants have reported weight loss from six to fifteen pounds. The unwanted weight comes off your body as you detox, eliminating toxins from your body. If losing weight is a concern for you, consider the modified version of the 12 Day Power Detox Program.

In addition to weight loss, you will also experience transformation in other areas of your life. You see, aside from the excess weight in pounds or kilograms, there are other weights we carry through stages of life from different incidences and experiences. Often, we have not identified these weights, but they are daily sabotaging our life. Therefore the 12 Day Power Detox Program is also a *spiritual journey* as you work on detoxing negative emotions; i.e. emotional baggage, burdens from the past or anything that's preventing you from being totally free.

The Program also provides the support and accountability needed to cheer you on to the finish line. The journey can get lonely at times and that extra support goes a long way.

At the end of the twelve days, you will have a healthier body with new healthy habits, a mind that's set to make healthy choices and a rejuvenated spirit. Imagine having a life which has rewards like fewer visits to the doctor, longer life, reduced medical expenses, happiness and increased energy. It's time to heal to your whole being. You can begin to live your best life if you act now.

THE BIRTH OF THE POWER DETOX PROGRAM

It was a beautiful day in the month of September. My day started off well in high spirits.

I listened to an audio message and made some declarations from Ephesians 3:20 which is one of my favorite scriptures.

> *"Now to Him who is able to [carry out His purpose and] do superabundantly more than all that we dare ask or think [infinitely beyond our greatest prayers, hopes, or dreams], according to His power that is at work within us."* Ephesians 3:20 AMP

I was enjoying being in God's presence as I meditated on the words of this verse. It felt like what is described in Ephesians 3:19.

> *"And [that you may come] to know [practically, through personal experience] the love of Christ which far surpasses [mere] knowledge [without experience], that you may be filled up [throughout your being] to all the fullness of God [so that you may have the richest experience of God's presence in your lives, completely filled and flooded with God Himself]."* **Ephesians 3:19 AMP**

I started getting more ideas for my business then I went to make my green smoothie still in my glory filled state. The smoothie I made was one of the recipes I was developing for the 12 Day Power Detox Program—the Apple Serenity Smoothie. I had a few sips and headed out to work, still feeling the presence of God. As I drove to work, I said to myself, "Today will be a good day to finish writing this detox program."

I got to work full of joy and giggles. While settling in, a lady coworker walked into my office and said she noticed I'd lost some weight recently. She sat down and ask what I was doing differently. She said she needed to lose weight in the next 3 weeks.

You see, I had put on a few pounds from holiday eating. I know... please don't judge me. This is what happens when you stuff your body with foods it's not used too. I had tried several things that worked for me in the past to lose the unwanted weight but it was not happening until I started drinking the green smoothies. My body needed a way to get rid of these unhealthy substances and the detox did it.

My coworker and I have had many talks about losing weight in the past, but I really didn't have something in writing to share with her, so I just gave her some weight loss tips. I told her about the detox program I was developing, and she said she wanted the details, so she could start the next day.

The good thing was, as I got the idea for the detox program, I started jotting down notes and creating recipes. Now in just a few hours, I was able to put it all together in a document that someone could follow.

During lunch, my coworker told another lady about the program and asked me to tell her about it. The other lady shared how she'd been stuck at a certain weight and wanted to lose a few more pounds.

So back to work, I finished up the nutrition part of the program during my lunch break and handed it over to them. I felt like a mom who just gave birth to a baby. I was excited to see them have results.

I was planning to launch the detox program that December as a gift to my fitness community, but I guess God had other plans.

It made me think about so many projects people want to start and never implement because of procrastination while there are people who need the idea to improve their lives.

The day continued and I started sharing this story with friends and family. Week by week, we had people starting the program and sharing their awesome results.

I typically try out a product or a program before I promote it, so I had to go through the detox program myself. Here are my observations each time I have completed the Detox Program.

It's like hitting a reset button. Each time I eat something after finishing the 12 Day Power Detox, I have to think about it and make the right choice. It made me think about how I want to spend my daily calories on what I'm eating. I felt clean on the inside, so I didn't want to eat any junk food.

I was able to get back into healthy habits like measuring my food portions, checking to see the correct serving size, and eating healthy snacks. I also craved healthier meals.

I lost 10 pounds the first time I completed the Program. I felt great overall and happier. People told me, "I looked younger. I had better concentration and focus. I drank the required daily intake of water and my digestive organs organs functioned better; i.e. bowel movements.

CHAPTER 1

THE ANATOMY OF A GREEN SMOOTHIE

BENEFITS OF GREEN SMOOTHIE DETOX

Our detox smoothie recipes are full of vitamins, antioxidants, fiber, and other healthy nutrients giving your body a detoxifying cleanse. They also contain large amounts of water, which helps to hydrate your body and boost metabolism.

I especially like the fact that you can get your daily dose of vitamins, minerals and other nutrients just in a one cup serving. People may not necessarily be open to trying a salad but are generally open to trying a cold cup of refreshing goodness.

Here are some benefits you'll experience over the next 12 days:

Cleanse your body: Over time there is a buildup of harmful toxins; preservatives, pesticides, heavy metals such as mercury and lead in the body through consumption of the food we eat and exposure to pollution. This can affect our metabolism, behavior, immune system, ultimately leading to disease.Our Detox Program is designed to stimulate the body to cleanse itself, helping the liver, kidneys and colon do what they naturally do to rid the body of toxins and waste.

Reduce the risk of serious diseases: It is well known that one way of preventing cancer and heart disease is to increase the number of fruits and vegetables in your diet. The more green smoothies you drink, the lower your risk.

Look younger: The increased fluids and power of natural foods in your diet will hydrate your skin and reduce your wrinkles making you look younger.

Feel energized: Fruits are a good source of energy but eaten alone will only provide short bursts of energy (they contain lots of sugars, which are quickly metabolized). Because of their high content of veggies, green smoothies have more balanced sugar content.

Weight loss: Increasing the number of fruits and vegetables you eat in a day gives your body an opportunity to shed excess fat and water weight built up from toxins stored in the body. Our green smoothies are low in calories but very filling. Because they contain high amounts of water and fiber, they'll make you feel as if you just ate a full meal. If you're trying to lose weight and belly fat, our green smoothies contain a combination of fruits and vegetables that will help fight hunger, reduce cravings and bloating while helping the pounds melt off easier. Even though this is not a weight loss program, participants who completed this program and reported their weight loss, have lost seven pounds to fifteen pounds in twelve days.

Crave less junk: When you increase the amount of healthy foods in your diet and decrease the unhealthy foods, you will naturally stop craving junk food and start craving more healthy food. You will begin a lifestyle of eating healthier even after completing the Detox Program.

Detox negative thoughts and emotions: Rejuvenate your soul and spirit by detoxing negative emotions with daily inspirational devotions. Negative emotions include anger, unforgiveness (offense), stress, worry and anxiety, fear, jealousy, pride, addiction, disappointment, failure, judgment, condemnation, betrayal, rejection and abandonment, harsh curse words and hate, etc.

Daniel Fast: This is one of the types of fasting based on how Daniel fasted in the Bible. During a Daniel Fast, you do not eat meat, dairy, sweets, fried food and bread. The only drink allowed is water. The goal is to eat healthy and natural, all unprocessed food items. Therefore, you get to try a variety of specified fruits, nuts, grains and vegetables. The smoothie recipes provided in our 12 Day Power Detox Program can be used as a part of the Daniel Fast Diet.

WHAT'S IN YOUR SMOOTHIE CUP?

Water: Water is essential for proper body function and circulation of nutrients in the body. It aids digestion of food by breaking it down so that your body can absorb the nutrients. Water flushes the liver tissues, aiding in the removal of toxins, and assists the kidneys during detox so the liver can focus on its own cleansing.

Vegetables: They are a good source of many nutrients, including iron, potassium, fiber, folate (folic acid) and vitamins.

Fruits: Fruits are important sources of many nutrients, including potassium, fiber, vitamin C and folate (folic acid). Fruits filled with antioxidants help the body fight diseases and cancers.

Plant-based protein and healthy fats: Nuts and seeds are good sources of fiber, heart-healthy fats, and provide a wide range of essential nutrients, including protein, vitamins and minerals such as calcium, iron, zinc, potassium, magnesium, and antioxidants.

HOW TO MAKE A DETOX SMOOTHIE

1. Add fresh green vegetables and water then blend.
2. Add fruits. Reduce the amount of water in the recipe and add ice if ALL the fruits used are fresh.
3. Add plant-based protein.
4. Blend until smooth and enjoy!

CHAPTER 2

PREPARING FOR THE DETOX PROGRAM

IMPORTANT NOTES

1. **Modified Detox Program:** You can ease into the Detox Program by doing the Modified Detox for Day 1 and 2. This allows you to have the smoothies for breakfast and dinner then have a healthy vegetable salad or soup (no meat or cheese and light dressing) for lunch. See **Sample Healthy Eating Recipes** section on page 52 for ideas.

2. **Snacking:** While on this program, you shouldn't feel hungry. If you feel hungry, eat one serving of the recommended healthy snacks between smoothie meals. One serving of raw nuts is about a handful. One serving of carrots is one cup.

3. **Measuring progress:** Weigh yourself first in the morning on Day 1, after using the bathroom. Take pictures of yourself and measurements of your chest, hip and waist before starting the 12 Day Power Detox Program. Record your measurements in a journal and date it. This will give you motivation as you see your weight drop day by day. Also, repeat the same measurements on Day 12.

4. **Exercise:** Do light or moderate intensity exercise daily for 30 minutes or at least 2.5 hours in a week.

5. **Stay hydrated – very important:** Stay hydrated by drinking water. Aim for at least eight cups of water per day totaling 64 ounces or four 16.9 ounce bottles. Add lemon to your water to make a powerful detox drink that will cleanse and alkalize your body.

6. **Detox tea:** Enjoy a detox tea of your choice all day. They help to improve liver function, as well as support the other digestive organs that play a role in detoxification. You can find a variety in the tea aisle of your grocery store.

7. **Rest:** Plan to get at least seven hours of sleep every night. The earlier you get to bed, the less you have to worry about getting hungry late at night. Sleep allows your body to rejuvenate and restore energy. Sleep aids the detox process and improves your emotional well-being.

   Studies have shown that a good night's sleep helps our brain regulate moods and prepares us for the next day's activities. Tissue growth and repair also occur during sleep. Growth hormones are released during sleep and hunger hormones are regulated. No wonder you may feel like eating high-calorie foods when you are sleep deprived.

8. **Bowel movements:** You will experience frequent bowel movements as a result of the detox process and drinking more water than you are used to, but it shouldn't be uncomfortable. It is important that you drink the recommended water intake to avoid dehydration. To avoid sleep disturbance, stop taking any liquid one or two hours before bedtime.

9. **Saltwater cleanse:** This gives your colon and digestive system a deeper cleanse by bringing on a forced bowel movement. Do the salt water cleanse on Week 1, Day 2 and Day 6, first thing in the morning on an empty stomach. Week 2 is optional and as needed. It is not recommended for everyone especially if you have health concerns.

To be honest, it is not a pleasant experience. It's only for the daring ones. It is very important to drink water throughout the day if you are doing the salt water cleanse to avoid dehydration. Mix 4 cups (32 oz.) of warm water with 2 level teaspoons of unrefined sea salt in a container. Shake well, and then drink the entire container of salt water. It should work as long as you don't use iodized table salt. Plan to stay at home within the first two or three hours of drinking the salt water.

10. **Detox bath soaking:** Your skin is your largest organ and one of the primary organs of elimination. A detox bath will help you eliminate toxins through your skin. Fill the bathtub with warm water. Dissolve Epsom salt, baking soda and your favorite essential oils in bath water. Soak in bath water for at least thirty minutes or as long as desired. Play some soothing music in the background that helps you stay calm, relaxed and takes you to a happy place.

11. **Consult your doctor:** If you have any existing medical conditions, always consult your doctor before beginning any diet or exercise program. If at any time you feel you are not able to continue the full cleanse due to any kind of discomfort, please switch to the Modified Detox Program or stop the Program.

PREP WEEK

The prep week is the week before you start the 12 Day Power Detox Program. It should be spent doing all the activities listed in the Checklist below. Review and complete these action items.

PREP WEEK CHECKLIST

1. Read the **Important Notes** and **F.A.Q.** sections on pages 20 and 25, the rest of this book using the Table of Contents as a guide to view important sections.
2. Take pictures of yourself and measurements of your chest, hip and waist before you begin the Detox Program.
3. Clean out any junk food in the food pantry or cabinet, fridge and freezer at home and at work. Removing anything you won't be eating during the twelve days will help reduce the temptation to break your detox and prevent you from immediately going back to eating them after the Detox Program.
4. Bookmark the Meal and Activity Plan (M.A.P.) on pages 36 and 37. You will be referring to it frequently.
5. Schedule time to do your grocery shopping with the list provided and plan out your meals and activities using the M.A.P. provided for Week 1 and 2.
6. Pack the daily recipe food items and snacks in freezer bags for the first six days and store in the freezer. Fresh fruits like bananas can be peeled and cut into slices. Place the banana slices into freezer bags or container before freezing. This also applies to most fresh fruits and makes it easy to prepare your smoothies in the morning.
7. Free up and schedule the time to exercise 30 minutes for five days each week. Rest for two days to allow your muscles to recover and rebuild. Please refer to the M.A.P.
8. Schedule time every morning to read the 12 Day Power Detox Devotion. Set a reminder on your alarm or calendar.
9. Join the Private Facebook Support Group. Search for "12 Day Power Detox."
10. Get a journal to record your 12-Day experience.

GROCERY LIST

Below is your grocery list for Week 1. Repeat this list for Week 2 as needed. You can find most of the groceries listed at a health food store near you. As your budget allows, buy organic produce. Choosing organic produce lowers your exposure to pesticides.

The Power Green Mix is a combination of two or more of the following fresh vegetables; spinach, kale or swiss chard. If you don't find a prepackaged bag at the grocery store, you can buy individual bags and make your own mix using equal portions. Spring Mix Greens usually come prepackaged in the store.

For Green Smoothie beginners, you can start off with spinach as the only green in the smoothie for the first two days, then add variety by the third day.

Use one or a combination of two of the plant-based protein and healthy fats like flaxseed meal, chia seeds, pumpkin seeds, hemp seeds and unsalted almond butter. Flaxseed meal is recommended for starters.

1. 15 ounces (oz.) of Power Green Mix (Bag contains a mix of fresh green vegetables, i.e. spinach, chard, and kale)
2. 10 ounces (oz.) of Spring Mix Greens (Fresh Vegetables)
3. 3 medium size and 1 small size apple, i.e. Gala or any red apple of your choice (cored and cut into pieces)
4. 1 small size Green or Granny Smith apple
5. 3 small or 2 large size bananas. Buy medium ripe if available.
6. 1 medium size pear (Use pear as a substitute for bananas and apples as you desire)
7. 10 ounces (oz.) of frozen or 1 medium size fresh pineapple
8. 10 ounces (oz.) of frozen or 1 medium size fresh mango
9. 10 ounces (oz.) of frozen or 3 medium size fresh peaches
10. 10 ounces (oz.) of frozen or fresh mixed berries, i.e. a combination of two or more of the following: strawberries, raspberries, blackberries and blueberries.
11. 10 ounces (oz.) of frozen or fresh blueberries
12. 10 ounces (oz.) of frozen or fresh strawberries
13. 1 pack of unsweetened frozen acai berry purees (3.5 oz.). Week 1 Recipe for Triple Berry Love Smoothie (Option 1). If the acai berry puree packs are not available, use the Week 2, Option 2 recipe.

14. 1 bunch of grapes
15. 6 lemons (Add to drinking water daily.)
16. Uniodized sea salt
17. Snacks: See the **Snack** section on page 46 for a list of Preferred Snacks. Pick about four snacks, i.e. 2 vegetables, 1 low sugar fruit and a variety of nuts.
18. Plant-based protein and healthy fat, like flaxseed meal, chia seeds, pumpkin seeds, hemp seeds and unsalted almond butter.
19. Detox tea of your choice. If Detox tea is not available, you can use any one of the following: Green Tea, Ginger Tea or Peppermint Tea.

OTHER ITEMS NEEDED

1. 2-Cup measuring cup or a set with several sizes.
2. A set of measuring spoons with several sizes.
3. 3 water bottles or cups with straws (14-15 ounces), BPA Free recommended.
4. Blender. I prefer Oster® but use what you have and like.
5. Journal – Use this to record your observations, results, weight, measurements and devotion notes.

FOODS TO AVOID ON THE DETOX PROGRAM

Dairy: All including butter, cheese, cream, milk, and yogurt.

Butter and mayonnaise: All.

Grains: All includingwheat, corn, barley, rye, brown rice, oats, whole-wheat pasta or crackers. Most oats (oats are usually contaminated with gluten unless you can find a gluten-free brand).

Fruits and vegetables: Oranges, juices, corn, creamed vegetables.

Animal protein: Pork, beef, veal, sausage, cold cuts, canned meats, frankfurters, shellfish.

Nuts and seeds: Peanuts.

Oils: Shortening, processed oils, high-calorie salad dressings, spreads and fried foods.

Drinks: Alcohol, caffeinated beverages, and soft drinks.

Sweeteners: All except stevia. Avoid white and brown refined sugars, honey, maple syrup, high-fructose corn syrup, and evaporated cane juice.

All refined & processed food products: Artificial flavorings, chemicals, food additives, preservatives, white flour, and white rice.

Bread and baked goods: All types.

Condiments: chocolate, ketchup, relish, chutney, barbecue sauce, and teriyaki.

FREQUENTLY ASKED QUESTIONS (F.A.Q.)

Why should I detox my spirit, soul and body?
EVERYONE needs to detox. You breathe polluted air, you experience stress, both of which cause physical problems in the body. Pollutants such as ozone irritate breathing, trigger asthma symptoms and cause lung and heart diseases. Stress increases cholesterol levels in the body.

No person's diet is perfect. If you can answer this question honestly and your answer is "Yes," then you probably don't need to do a detox. Are you willing to guarantee that you eat a healthy meal plan that is void of processed foods, genetically modified foods, caffeine, food coloring, refined sugars, alcohol or pesticides?

Think of your body as a vehicle requiring regular maintenance like an oil change. Routine oil and filter changes help remove particles and sludge, keeping engines at peak condition. Buildup from dirty oil robs a vehicle's fuel economy and power and makes internal components work harder. An engine that works too hard will end up having more problems down the road, as well as a shorter lifespan.

The organs of your body work like the engine of a vehicle. Regular maintenance and detox are necessary to keep your body in good health thereby prolonging your life.

As you may know, man is a 3 part being with a spirit, soul and body. Your soul is the dimension of man which deals with the mental realm. It consists of the mind, will and emotions. It's the part that reasons and thinks. The emotions are the responses (feelings) to the information which comes to us from the physical world around us and from the spirit within us. We respond to emotions by crying or feeling like crying over news that we hear with our ears, but we can also cry when, from our spirit, we become aware of how much God loves us. The soul has not only the memory of things in your life which have happened but the way you felt about those things in your emotions.

The 12 Day Power Detox Devotional will guide you through the process of detoxing negative emotions from your soul that you've experienced while embracing positive emotions. You will begin to feel happier, free to love and trust again.

I'm skeptical about adding green vegetables to my smoothies, what do you recommend?

For Green Smoothie beginners, you can start off with spinach as the only greens in the smoothie for the first two days, and then add variety by the 3rd day. Start with 2 cups of spinach and add the other ingredients. After blending, taste before you add more green vegetables.

How is this program different from any other detox or cleanse program?

This program offers a unique and holistic approach to detoxing. It has the Nutrition and Wellness components which will help you *revive, restore and rejuvenate your spirit, soul and body.*

Variety is the spice of life. Over the next 12 days, you get to try different kinds of fruits, nuts and vegetables which will supercharge your body.

I'm worried about losing any more weight but I still want to try the Detox Program, what should I do?

Do the Modified Detox Program. Drink the Green Smoothies for breakfast and dinner, eat vegetarian salad or soup for lunch and snack in between meals.

How do I complete the Detox Program successfully?

To have a successful completion, you need to follow the smoothie recipes and the M.A.P (Meal and Activity Plan), be disciplined, determined, have support and accountability.

If this is your first time doing a vegetarian meal plan, it is okay to start with the Modified 12 Day Power Detox Program. Read the **Important Notes** section on page 20 and the rest of this book using the Table of Contents as a guide to view important sections.

Complete the action items listed in the **Prep Week** on page 22. Pack the daily recipe food items and snacks in freezer bags for the first 6 days during the Prep Week. Keep the 12 Day Power Detox Meal Plan in a visible part of your home or office as a reminder throughout the day.

How do I get accountability and support to keep me going on this Program?

Join the Private Facebook Support Group. Search for "12 Day Power Detox." This is where you will get the support and accountability you need from Coach Ade and other participants who will cheer you on to the finish line.

What should I do if I feel hungry during the Detox?

During this program, you shouldn't be hungry if you follow the meal plans for Week 1 and 2. When you feel hungry, eat one serving of the recommended healthy snacks between smoothie meals. One serving of raw nuts is about a handful. One serving of baby carrots is 1 cup. Make sure you are drinking 64 ounces of water daily and sipping your Detox Tea as well.

This program is too much of a challenge, I feel like quitting?

Before you throw in the towel, switch to the Modified Detox Program for as long as you can. The food cravings will always show up; the temptations at work, home or at a get-together. If you slip and ate something outside of what's recommended on this Detox Program, the decision to continue depends on you. You can pick up the next day or choose to start over at another time. Your results will vary from participants who followed the meal plan and completed the Detox Program.

How long can I stay on the 12 Day Power Detox?

If you are going to keep drinking the smoothie recipes as part of your regular healthy meal plan, rotate your greens. Try a variety of fresh green vegetables in your smoothie. We recommend that you do not stay on the 12 Day Power Detox program longer than 2 weeks at a time unless you are doing the Modified Detox Program or as part of the Daniel Fast which allows you add more protein to your diet. You can repeat it periodically throughout the year, for example every 3 months.

What should I do if I experience any of the following?

Headaches: Headaches are one of the common side effects of detoxing your body. It may be a dull, prolonged headache. This usually happens within the first few days of the detox, especially for first-timers. Sudden withdrawal from caffeine, sugar, drinking alcohol, smoking or processed foods, can have this effect, as can dehydration. It is not recommended that you take pain relief medications during the detox. The most effective treatment for headaches during a detox is still to drink plenty of water as recommended and get some rest.

Cravings or Hunger Pangs: You may experience hunger pangs the first few days of the detox but it will eventually stop after a few days as the body successfully acclimates. Over time, the Green Smoothies will help you eliminate cravings but you may have craving for different food items initially.

Here are a few tips to overcome your cravings or hunger pangs, drink a bottle of water or detox tea; go for a walk or have a nap; eat a handful of nuts or your favorite vegetable; change the focus by doing your favorite activity or exercise. During the Detox, sometimes I feel like chewing on something, so I would grab one serving of baby carrots and drink water. This really helps!

Constipation/Diarrhea: Participants who follow the recipes and instructions typically do not experience these symptoms but there could be exceptions. Green Smoothies are high in fiber so digestion should improve. Once your body adjusts to the increase in healthy food and fiber, the symptoms will subside–usually within a couple of days. Constipation may be due to the sudden increase of fiber in the diet. Check your water intake. If you haven't had the specified 64 ounces, drink up. Also make sure you are following the measurements on the recipes.

The Salt Water Cleanse is also a good way to get rid of constipation if the other suggested methods fail. See the **Important Notes** section on page 20.

Breakouts: Your skin is the largest detox organ and it helps your body release toxins through your pores in the form of sweat. If you experience breakouts, it's probably because of the detox and it should clear up in a few days.

Important: If any of the above symptoms persist beyond a week, then they may signal a necessary change that you need to make. Please stop the Detox Program and consult your doctor.

CHAPTER 3

THE PROGRAM

SMOOTHIE RECIPES

There are six delicious recipes provided for you. If you're not satisfied with the taste of one of the six recipes you can always switch it out with another one, but don't let that stop you from completing the Detox Program. You have a variety of recipes to choose from. Put as much fresh green vegetables as you can in one cup.

Feel free to add more water and fresh green vegetables to your smoothie as you desire. Don't be tempted to add more fruit especially if you're fighting a sugar craving or addiction. You can use fresh or frozen fruits. If you use fresh fruits, peel and core if necessary, cut into pieces and add ice.

SMOOTHIE MEAL PORTIONS
Each smoothie recipe contains three servings. Divide the blended smoothie into three portions. Enjoy smoothies for breakfast, lunch and dinner for ten days. On Day 11 and 12, begin to transition into regular healthy clean eating. By the thirteenth day, you should be ready to eat other food items but strive to make healthy choices. You can also continue to enjoy the green smoothies either as a breakfast or dinner meal.

WEEK 1 SMOOTHIE RECIPES

DAY 1 – Tropical Paradise Smoothie
3 cups of Power Greens Mix
2 cups of water
1 medium size apple (cored and cut into pieces)
1 cup of frozen or fresh cut pineapple
½ cup of frozen or fresh cut mango
2 tablespoons of plant-based protein

DAY 2 – Heavenly Green Joy Smoothie
3 cups of Power Green Mix
2 cups of water
1 medium size apple (cored and cut into pieces)
½ cup of frozen or fresh cut pineapple
½ cup of frozen or fresh strawberries
½ cup of grapes (optional)
2 tablespoons of plant-based protein

DAY 3 – Holy Bananas Smoothie

3 cups of Power Greens Mix
2 cups of water
2 small size bananas or 1 large banana (medium ripe)
½ cup of frozen or fresh cut peach
½ cup of frozen or fresh cut pineapple
2 tablespoons of plant-based protein

DAY 4 – Triple Berry Love Smoothie (Option 1)

3 cups of Spring Mix Greens
2 cups of water
1 cup of frozen or fresh blueberries
½ cup of frozen or fresh strawberries
1 pack of unsweetened frozen acai berry puree (3.5 oz)
1 medium size pear (cored and cut into pieces)
2 tablespoons of plant-based protein

DAY 5 – Apple Serenity Smoothie

3 cups of Spring Mix Greens
2 cups of water
1 small size green or Granny Smith apple (cored and cut into pieces)
1 small size apple i.e. Gala or any red apple (cored and cut into pieces)
½ cup of fresh or frozen strawberries
½ cup of fresh or frozen blueberries
2 tablespoons of plant-based protein

DAY 6 – Berry Delight Smoothie*

3 cups of Power Greens Mix
2 cups of water
1 medium size apple (cored and cut into pieces)
2 cups of fresh or frozen mixed berries
2 tablespoons of plant-based protein

This smoothie may require additional blending time to make sure the berry seeds are properly blended.

DAY 7 – Tropical Paradise Smoothie

3 cups of Power Greens Mix
2 cups of water
1 medium size apple (cored and cut into pieces)
1 cup of frozen or fresh cut pineapple
½ cup of frozen or fresh cut mango
2 tablespoons of plant-based protein

WEEK 2 SMOOTHIE RECIPES

DAY 8 – Apple Serenity Smoothie
3 cups of Spring Mix Greens
2 cups of water
1 small size green or Granny Smith apple (cored and cut into pieces)
1 small size apple i.e. Gala or any red apple (cored and cut into pieces)
½ cup of fresh or frozen strawberries
½ cup of fresh or frozen blueberries
2 tablespoons of plant-based protein

DAY 9 – Triple Berry Love Smoothie (Option 2)
3 cups of Spring Mix Greens
2 cups of water
1 cup of frozen or fresh blueberries
½ cup of frozen or fresh strawberries
½ cup of grapes
1 small size banana
2 tablespoons of plant-based protein

DAY 10 – Holy Bananas Smoothie
3 cups of Power Greens Mix
2 cups of water
2 small size bananas or 1 large banana (medium ripe)
½ cup of frozen or fresh cut peach
½ cup of frozen or fresh cut pineapple
2 tablespoons of plant-based protein

DAY 11 – Breakfast and Dinner: Heavenly Green Joy Smoothie
2 cups of Power Green Mix
1½ cups of water
1 medium size apple (cored and cut into pieces)
½ cup of frozen or fresh cut pineapple
½ cup of frozen or fresh strawberries
½ cup of grapes (*optional*)
2 tablespoons of plant-based protein

Lunch: Enjoy a healthy salad with a mix of vegetables, fruits and nuts.

DAY 12 – Breakfast: Berry Delight Smoothie*

2 cups of Power Greens Mix
1½ cups of water
1 medium size apple (cored and cut into pieces)
1 cup of frozen or fresh mixed berries
2 tablespoons of plant-based protein

* *This smoothie may require additional blending time to make sure the berries seeds are properly blended.*

Lunch: Enjoy a healthy salad with a mix of vegetables, fruits and nuts.
Dinner: Enjoy a healthy vegetable soup of your choice.

12 DAY POWER DETOX MEAL AND ACTIVITY PLAN (M.A.P)

First and Last Name:		Start Date:		Beginning Weight (lb.)
Allergies:	Favorite Smoothie Days		Weightloss at the end of the 12 Day Power Detox (lb.)	

DAY	BREAKFAST	SNACK	LUNCH	SNACK	DINNER	ACTIVITY
DAILY WATER INTAKE		1 Bottle - 16.9 fl.oz. + 1/2 Lemon		1 Bottle - 16.9 fl.oz.	1 Bottle - 16.9 fl.oz.	
WEEK 1						
MONDAY DAY 1	Tropical Paradise Smoothie	• Detox tea and **one serving of** • Raw or dry-roasted nuts (a handful) OR • Vegetables OR • Unsalted air popped popcorn	Tropical Paradise Smoothie Modified Detox: See Important Notes	• Detox tea and **one serving of** • Raw or dry-roasted nuts (a handful) OR • Vegetables OR • Unsalted air popped popcorn	Tropical Paradise Smoothie	Salt Water Cleanse: See Important Notes 30 mins of light or moderate intensity exercise
TUESDAY DAY 2	Heavenly Green Joy Smoothie	• Detox tea and **one serving of** • Raw or dry-roasted nuts (a handful) OR • Vegetables OR • Unsalted air popped popcorn	Heavenly Green Joy Smoothie	• Detox tea and **one serving of** • Raw or dry-roasted nuts (a handful) OR • Vegetables OR • Unsalted air popped popcorn	Heavenly Green Joy Smoothie	30 mins of light or moderate intensity exercise
WEDNESDAY DAY 3	Holy Bananas Smoothie	• Detox tea and **one serving of** • Raw or dry-roasted nuts (a handful) OR • Vegetables OR • Unsalted air popped popcorn	Holy Bananas Smoothie Modified Detox: See Important Notes	• Detox tea and **one serving of** • Raw or dry-roasted nuts (a handful) OR • Vegetables OR • Unsalted air popped popcorn	Holy Bananas Smoothie	30 mins of light or moderate intensity exercise
THURSDAY DAY 4	Triple Berry Love Smoothie (Option 1)	• Detox tea and **one serving of** • Raw or dry-roasted nuts (a handful) OR • Vegetables OR • Unsalted air popped popcorn	Triple Berry Love Smoothie (Option 1)	• Detox tea and **one serving of** • Raw or dry-roasted nuts (a handful) OR • Vegetables OR • Unsalted air popped popcorn	Triple Berry Love Smoothie (Option 1)	30 mins of light or moderate intensity exercise
FRIDAY DAY 5	Apple Serenity Smoothie	• Detox tea and **one serving of** • Raw or dry-roasted nuts (a handful) OR • Vegetables OR • Unsalted air popped popcorn	Apple Serenity Smoothie	• Detox tea and **one serving of** • Raw or dry-roasted nuts (a handful) OR • Vegetables OR • Unsalted air popped popcorn	Apple Serenity Smoothie	30 mins of light or moderate intensity exercise
SATURDAY DAY 6	Berry Delight Smoothie	• Detox tea and **one serving of** • Raw or dry-roasted nuts (a handful) OR • Vegetables OR • Unsalted air popped popcorn	Berry Delight Smoothie	• Detox tea and **one serving of** • Raw or dry-roasted nuts (a handful) OR • Vegetables OR • Unsalted air popped popcorn	Berry Delight Smoothie	Rest Day - Schedule time at the Spa/Sauna or Detox Bath Soaking

12 DAY POWER DETOX MEAL AND ACTIVITY PLAN (M.A.P)

DAY	BREAKFAST	SNACK	LUNCH	SNACK	DINNER	ACTIVITY
Allergies:		Favorite Smoothie Days		Weightloss at the end of the 12 Day Power Detox (lb.)		
DAILY WATER INTAKE		1 Bottle - 16.9 fl.oz. + 1/2 Lemon	1 Bottle - 16.9 fl.oz.	1 Bottle - 16.9 fl.oz. + 1/2 Lemon	1 Bottle - 16.9 fl.oz.	
SUNDAY DAY 7	Tropical Paradise Smoothie	Detox tea and **one serving of** ▲ Raw or dry-roasted nuts (a handful) OR ▲ Vegetables OR ▲ Unsalted air popped popcorn	Tropical Paradise Smoothie	Detox tea and **one serving of** ▲ Raw or dry-roasted nuts (a handful) OR ▲ Vegetables OR ▲ Unsalted air popped popcorn	Tropical Paradise Smoothie	Me Time - Detox Bath Soaking or Treat yourself to an activity you enjoy i.e. Manicure, Pedicure, Sleep etc.
MONDAY DAY 8	Apple Serenity Smoothie	Detox tea and **one serving of** ▲ Raw or dry-roasted nuts (a handful) OR ▲ Vegetables OR ▲ Unsalted air popped popcorn	Apple Serenity Smoothie	Detox tea and **one serving of** ▲ Raw or dry-roasted nuts (a handful) OR ▲ Vegetables OR ▲ Unsalted air popped popcorn	Apple Serenity Smoothie	30 mins of light or moderate intensity exercise
TUESDAY DAY 9	Triple Berry Love Smoothie (Option 2)	Detox tea and **one serving of** ▲ Raw or dry-roasted nuts (a handful) OR ▲ Vegetables OR ▲ Unsalted air popped popcorn	Triple Berry Love Smoothie (Option 2)	Detox tea and **one serving of** ▲ Raw or dry-roasted nuts (a handful) OR ▲ Vegetables OR ▲ Unsalted air popped popcorn	Triple Berry Love Smoothie (Option 2)	30 mins of light or moderate intensity exercise
WEDNESDAY DAY 10	Holy Bananas Smoothie	Detox tea and **one serving of** ▲ Raw or dry-roasted nuts (a handful) OR ▲ Vegetables OR ▲ Unsalted air popped popcorn	Holy Bananas Smoothie	Detox tea and **one serving of** ▲ Raw or dry-roasted nuts (a handful) OR ▲ Vegetables OR ▲ Unsalted air popped popcorn	Holy Bananas Smoothie	30 mins of light or moderate intensity exercise
THURSDAY DAY 11	Heavenly Green Joy Smoothie	Detox tea and **one serving of** ▲ Raw or dry-roasted nuts (a handful) OR ▲ Vegetables OR ▲ Unsalted air popped popcorn	Heavenly Green Joy Smoothie	Detox tea and **one serving of** ▲ Raw or dry-roasted nuts (a handful) OR ▲ Vegetables OR ▲ Unsalted air popped popcorn	Heavenly Green Joy Smoothie	30 mins of light or moderate intensity exercise
FRIDAY DAY 12	Berry Delight Smoothie	Detox tea and **one serving of** ▲ Raw or dry-roasted nuts (a handful) OR ▲ Vegetables OR ▲ Unsalted air popped popcorn	Berry Delight Smoothie	Detox tea and **one serving of** ▲ Raw or dry-roasted nuts (a handful) OR ▲ Vegetables OR ▲ Unsalted air popped popcorn	Berry Delight Smoothie	30 mins of light or moderate intensity exercise
SATURDAY DAY 13	Tropical Paradise Smoothie	Healthy Snack	Healthy Lunch	Healthy Snack	Healthy Dinner	30 mins of light or moderate intensity exercise

W
E
E
K
2

TROPICAL SMOOTHIE RECIPES

The recipes in this section were specially created for people living in tropical countries around the world.

Tropical fruits are grown and developed in high-temperature climatic zones, covering most of the tropical and subtropical areas of Asia, Africa, Central America, South America, the Caribbean and Oceania. Pomegranates, mangoes, papayas, avocados, bananas, pineapples, guavas, kiwis and passion fruit are some popular examples. These fruits are a primary source of nutrition and a delicious component of a healthy, balanced diet. The combination of the fruits chosen for the tropical recipes is nutritious and tasty.

Here are a few suggestions to keep in mind while making your delicious cup of tropical goodness. Cucumber can be used, peeled or unpeeled, depending on your preference. For a colder and smoother smoothie, keep fruits frozen. You will use less ice which means a less diluted drink. It's also a great way to prevent overripened fruits.

PREP WEEK

The prep week is the week before you start the 12 Day Power Detox Program. It should be spent doing all the activities listed in the Checklist below. Review and complete these action items.

PREP WEEK CHECKLIST

1. Read the **Important Notes** and **F.A.Q.** sections on pages 20 and 25, the rest of this book using the Table of Contents as a guide to view important sections.
2. Take pictures of yourself and measurements of your chest, hip and waist before you begin the Detox Program.
3. Clean out any junk food in the food pantry or cabinet, fridge and freezer at home and at work. Removing anything you won't be eating during the twelve days will help reduce the temptation to break your detox and prevent you from immediately going back to eating them after the Detox Program.
4. Bookmark the Meal and Activity Plan (M.A.P.) on pages 44 and 45.

You will be referring to it frequently.

5. Schedule time to do your grocery shopping with the list provided and plan out your meals and activities using the M.A.P. provided for Week 1 and 2. You will be referring to it frequently.

6. Pack the daily recipe food items and snacks in freezer bags for the first six days and store in the freezer. Fresh fruits like bananas can be peeled and cut into slices. Place the banana slices into freezer bags or container before freezing. This also applies to most fresh fruits and makes it easy to prepare your smoothies in the morning.

7. Free up and schedule the time to exercise 30 minutes for five days each week. Rest for two days to allow your muscles to recover and rebuild. Please refer to the M.A.P.

8. Schedule time every morning to read the 12 Day Power Detox Devotion. Set a reminder on your alarm or calendar.

9. Join the Private Facebook Support Group. Search for "12 Day Power Detox."

10. Get a journal to record your 12-Day experience.

GROCERY LIST

Below is your grocery list for Week 1. Repeat this list for Week 2 as needed. For Green Smoothie beginners, you can start off with spinach as the only greens in the smoothie for the first two days, and then add variety by the third day. Try a variety of fresh green vegetables available in your area. Use one or a combination of two of the plant-based protein and healthy fats e.g. flaxseed meal, chia seeds, pumpkin seeds, hemp seeds and unsalted almond butter. Flaxseed meal is recommended for starters.

1. 25 ounces (oz.) or 1 kilogram of fresh green vegetables e.g. spinach and chard.
2. 5 medium size apples (cored and cut into pieces). Use green apples if available.
3. 2 small or 1 large size green bananas. Buy medium ripe if available.
4. 1 medium size pear (Use pear as a substitute for bananas and apples as you desire)
5. 1 medium size pineapple
6. 1 medium size mango
7. 1 medium size papaya

8. 1 medium size watermelon
9. 1 medium size cucumbers
10. 1 bunch of grapes
11. 6 lemons (Add to drinking water daily.)
12. Uniodized sea salt
13. Snacks: See **Snack** section on page 46 for a list of preferred snacks. Pick about four snacks i.e. 2 vegetables, 1 low sugar fruit and a variety of nuts.
14. Plant-based protein and healthy fat e.g. flaxseed meal, chia seeds, pumpkin seeds, hemp seeds, unsalted almond butter.
15. Green Tea, Ginger Tea or Peppermint Tea.

OTHER ITEMS NEEDED

1. 2-Cup measuring cup or a set with several sizes. You can use a teacup if measuring cups are not available.
2. A set of measuring spoons with several sizes.
3. 3 water bottles or cups with straws (14–15 ounces), BPA Free recommended.
4. Blender.
5. Journal – Use this to record your observations, results, weight, measurements and devotion notes.

WEEK 1 SMOOTHIE RECIPES

DAY 1 – Tropical Paradise Smoothie
3 cups/handfuls of spinach
2 cups of water
1 medium size apple (cored and cut into pieces)
1 cup of frozen or fresh cut pineapple
½ cup of frozen or fresh cut mango
2 tablespoons of plant-based protein

DAY 2 – Pineapple Heaven Smoothie
3 cups/handfuls of spinach
2 cups of water
1 medium size apple (cored and cut into pieces)
1 cup of frozen or fresh cut pineapple
1 cup of frozen or fresh cut watermelon
2 tablespoons of plant-based protein

DAY 3 – Holy Bananas Smoothie*
3 cups/handfuls of spinach
2 cups of water
2 small or 1 large size, medium ripe bananas
½ medium size cucumber* (cut into slices)
½ cup of frozen or fresh cut pineapple
2 tablespoons of plant-based protein
* *Try blending the cucumber peeled and unpeeled. The skin of cucumbers has some great benefits but ultimately make the smoothie to your taste.*

DAY 4 – Merry Mango Smoothie
3 cups/handfuls of spinach
2 cups of water
1 cup of frozen or fresh cut mango
½ medium size cucumber (cut into slices)
1 medium size green apple (cored and cut into pieces)
2 tablespoons of plant-based protein

DAY 5 – Mellow Green Smoothie
3 cups/handfuls of spinach
2 cups of water
1 medium size apple (cored and cut into pieces)
1 cup of frozen or fresh cut watermelon
1 cup of frozen or fresh cut mango
2 tablespoons of plant-based protein

DAY 6 – Papa's Delight Smoothie
3 cups/handfuls of spinach
2 cups of water
1 medium size apple (cored and cut into pieces)
1 cup of frozen or fresh cut papaya (pawpaw)
1 cup of frozen or fresh cut watermelon
½ cup of grapes (optional)
2 tablespoons of plant-based protein

DAY 7 – Tropical Paradise Smoothie
3 cups/handfuls of spinach
2 cups of water
1 medium size apple (cored and cut into pieces)
1 cup of frozen or fresh cut pineapple
½ cup of frozen or fresh cut mango
2 tablespoons of plant-based protein

WEEK 2 SMOOTHIE RECIPES

DAY 8 – Pineapple Heaven Smoothie
3 cups/handfuls of spinach
2 cups of water
1 medium size apple (cored and cut into pieces)
1 cup of frozen or fresh cut pineapple
1 cup of frozen or fresh cut watermelon
2 tablespoons of plant-based protein

DAY 9 – Merry Mango Smoothie
3 cups/handfuls of spinach
2 cups of water
1 cup of frozen or fresh cut mango
½ medium size cucumber (cut into slices)
1 medium size green apple (cored and cut into pieces)
2 tablespoons of plant-based protein

DAY 10 – Holy Bananas Smoothie
3 cups/handfuls of spinach
2 cups of water
2 small or 1 large size, medium ripe bananas
½ medium size cucumber (cut into slices)
½ cup of frozen or fresh cut pineapple
2 tablespoons of plant-based protein

DAY 11 – Breakfast and Dinner: Mellow Green Smoothie
2 cups/handfuls of spinach
1½ cups of water
1 medium size apple (cored and cut into pieces)
½ cup of frozen or fresh cut watermelon
½ cup of frozen or fresh cut mango
2 tablespoons of plant-based protein

Dinner: Enjoy a healthy vegetable soup of your choice.

DAY 12 Breakfast: Papa's Delight Smoothie

2 cups/handfuls of spinach
1 cup of water
1 medium size apple (cored and cut into pieces)
½ cup of frozen or fresh cut papaya(pawpaw)
½ cup of frozen or fresh cut watermelon
½ cup of grapes (optional)
2 tablespoons of plant-based protein

Lunch: Enjoy a healthy salad with a mix of vegetables, fruits and nuts.
Dinner: Enjoy a healthy vegetable soup of your choice.

TROPICAL - 12 DAY POWER DETOX MEAL AND ACTIVITY PLAN (M.A.P)

First and Last Name: Start Date: Beginning Weight (Ib.)

Allergies: Favorite Smoothie Days   Weight loss at the end of the 12 Day Power Detox (Ib.)

DAY	BREAKFAST	SNACK	LUNCH	SNACK	DINNER	ACTIVITY
DAILY WATER INTAKE		1 Bottle - 16.9 fl.oz. + $^{1}/_{2}$ Lemon		1 Bottle - 16.9 fl.oz.	1 Bottle - 16.9 fl.oz. + $^{1}/_{2}$ Lemon	1 Bottle - 16.9 fl.oz.
MONDAY DAY 1	Tropical Paradise Smoothie	▸ Detox tea and **one serving of** ▸ Raw or dry-roasted nuts (a handful) OR ▸ Vegetables OR ▸ Unsalted air popped popcorn	Tropical Paradise Smoothie Modified Detox: See Important Notes	▸ Detox tea and **one serving of** ▸ Raw or dry-roasted nuts (a handful) OR ▸ Vegetables OR ▸ Unsalted air popped popcorn	Tropical Paradise Smoothie	30 mins of light or moderate intensity exercise
TUESDAY DAY 2	Pineapple Heaven Smoothie	▸ Detox tea and **one serving of** ▸ Raw or dry-roasted nuts (a handful) OR ▸ Vegetables OR ▸ Unsalted air popped popcorn	Pineapple Heaven Smoothie Modified Detox: See Important Notes	▸ Detox tea and **one serving of** ▸ Raw or dry-roasted nuts (a handful) OR ▸ Vegetables OR ▸ Unsalted air popped popcorn	Pineapple Heaven Smoothie	30 mins of light or moderate intensity exercise
WEDNESDAY DAY 3	Holy Bananas Smoothie	▸ Detox tea and **one serving of** ▸ Raw or dry-roasted nuts (a handful) OR ▸ Vegetables OR ▸ Unsalted air popped popcorn	Holy Bananas Smoothie	▸ Detox tea and **one serving of** ▸ Raw or dry-roasted nuts (a handful) OR ▸ Vegetables OR ▸ Unsalted air popped popcorn	Holy Bananas Smoothie	30 mins of light or moderate intensity exercise
THURSDAY DAY 4	Merry Mango Smoothie	▸ Detox tea and **one serving of** ▸ Raw or dry-roasted nuts (a handful) OR ▸ Vegetables OR ▸ Unsalted air popped popcorn	Merry Mango Smoothie	▸ Detox tea and **one serving of** ▸ Raw or dry-roasted nuts (a handful) OR ▸ Vegetables OR ▸ Unsalted air popped popcorn	Merry Mango Smoothie	30 mins of light or moderate intensity exercise
FRIDAY DAY 5	Mellow Green Smoothie	▸ Detox tea and **one serving of** ▸ Raw or dry-roasted nuts (a handful) OR ▸ Vegetables OR ▸ Unsalted air popped popcorn	Mellow Green Smoothie	▸ Detox tea and **one serving of** ▸ Raw or dry-roasted nuts (a handful) OR ▸ Vegetables OR ▸ Unsalted air popped popcorn	Mellow Green Smoothie	30 mins of light or moderate intensity exercise
SATURDAY DAY 6	Papa's Delight Smoothie	▸ Detox tea and **one serving of** ▸ Raw or dry-roasted nuts (a handful) OR ▸ Vegetables OR ▸ Unsalted air popped popcorn	Papa's Delight Smoothie	▸ Detox tea and **one serving of** ▸ Raw or dry-roasted nuts (a handful) OR ▸ Vegetables OR ▸ Unsalted air popped popcorn	Papa's Delight Smoothie	Rest Day - Schedule time at the Spa/Sauna or Detox Bath Soaking
						Salt Water Cleanse: See Important Notes

W E E K 1

TROPICAL - 12 DAY POWER DETOX MEAL AND ACTIVITY PLAN (M.A.P)

Allergies:		Favorite Smoothie Days		Weightloss at the end of the 12 Day Power Detox (lb.)		
DAY	**BREAKFAST**	**SNACK**	**LUNCH**	**SNACK**	**DINNER**	**ACTIVITY**
DAILY WATER INTAKE		1 Bottle - 16.9 fl.oz. + 1/2 Lemon	1 Bottle - 16.9 fl.oz.	1 Bottle - 16.9 fl.oz. + 1/2 Lemon	1 Bottle - 16.9 fl.oz.	
SUNDAY DAY 7	Tropical Paradise Smoothie	Detox tea and **one serving of** ▸ Raw or dry-roasted nuts (a handful) OR ▸ Vegetables OR ▸ Unsalted air popped popcorn	Tropical Paradise Smoothie	Detox tea and **one serving of** ▸ Raw or dry-roasted nuts (a handful) OR ▸ Vegetables OR ▸ Unsalted air popped popcorn	Tropical Paradise Smoothie	Me Time - Detox Bath Soaking or Treat yourself to an activity you enjoy i.e Manicure, Pedicure, Sleep etc.
MONDAY DAY 8	Pineapple Heaven Smoothie	Detox tea and **one serving of** ▸ Raw or dry-roasted nuts (a handful) OR ▸ Vegetables OR ▸ Unsalted air popped popcorn	Pineapple Heaven Smoothie	Detox tea and **one serving of** ▸ Raw or dry-roasted nuts (a handful) OR ▸ Vegetables OR ▸ Unsalted air popped popcorn	Pineapple Heaven Smoothie	30 mins of light or moderate intensity exercise
TUESDAY DAY 9	Merry Mango Smoothie	Detox tea and **one serving of** ▸ Raw or dry-roasted nuts (a handful) OR ▸ Vegetables OR ▸ Unsalted air popped popcorn	Merry Mango Smoothie	Detox tea and **one serving of** ▸ Raw or dry-roasted nuts (a handful) OR ▸ Vegetables OR ▸ Unsalted air popped popcorn	Merry Mango Smoothie	30 mins of light or moderate intensity exercise
WEDNESDAY DAY 10	Holy Bananas Smoothie	Detox tea and **one serving of** ▸ Raw or dry-roasted nuts (a handful) OR ▸ Vegetables OR ▸ Unsalted air popped popcorn	Holy Bananas Smoothie	Detox tea and **one serving of** ▸ Raw or dry-roasted nuts (a handful) OR ▸ Vegetables OR ▸ Unsalted air popped popcorn	Holy Bananas Smoothie	30 mins of light or moderate intensity exercise
THURSDAY DAY 11	Mellow Green Smoothie	Detox tea and **one serving of** ▸ Raw or dry-roasted nuts (a handful) OR ▸ Vegetables OR ▸ Unsalted air popped popcorn	Mellow Green Smoothie	Detox tea and **one serving of** ▸ Raw or dry-roasted nuts (a handful) OR ▸ Vegetables OR ▸ Unsalted air popped popcorn	Mellow Green Smoothie	30 mins of light or moderate intensity exercise
FRIDAY DAY 12	Papa's Delight Smoothie	Detox tea and **one serving of** ▸ Raw or dry-roasted nuts (a handful) OR ▸ Vegetables OR ▸ Unsalted air popped popcorn	Papa's Delight Smoothie	Detox tea and **one serving of** ▸ Raw or dry-roasted nuts (a handful) OR ▸ Vegetables OR ▸ Unsalted air popped popcorn	Papa's Delight Smoothie	30 mins of light or moderate intensity exercise
SATURDAY DAY 13	Tropical Paradise Smoothie	Healthy Snack	Healthy Lunch	Healthy Snack	Healthy Dinner	30 mins of light or moderate intensity exercise

WEEK 2

SNACKS

I recommend eating nuts and vegetables as a snack since you already have fruits in your smoothies. My preferred snacks are baby carrots, celery sticks, cucumber, jicama and a variety of raw or dry- roasted nuts. Below is a list of other snacks you can choose from.

Raw or dry-roasted nuts: Nuts with no added salt or sugar and not cooked in oil. Eat a variety of raw nuts e.g. walnuts, almonds, macadamia nuts, hazelnuts, pecans, Brazil, pistachio etc.

Raw vegetables and fruits: Enjoy a variety of vegetables; carrots, celery sticks, cucumber, jicama etc. And low sugar fruits; raspberries, strawberries, blackberries, kiwis, grapefruit, avocado, cantaloupe, guava, etc.

Unsalted air popped popcorn

SPICE UP YOUR SMOOTHIE

You can add flavor to your smoothie by adding one or a combination of these ingredients. Various spices enhance both flavor and nutrition. Experiment with them and perfect the taste. Cinnamon, cayenne pepper, ginger, and nutmeg, are a few good options.

FRESH GINGER
Fresh ginger adds a distinct peppery flavor to smoothies and balances out the sweet flavor of fresh fruit. Try adding about a teaspoon of grated fresh ginger per serving of smoothie. It blends well with pears and strawberries.

Ginger has so many health benefits, including anti-inflammatory properties, blood sugar regulation, and gastrointestinal relief. It may be best known for helping relieve nausea related to seasickness, chemotherapy-related nausea, nausea after surgery, and morning sickness. Ginger may also help protect against osteoarthritis because of its anti-inflammatory properties.

When eaten raw, ginger has a very spicy flavor. A little caution, due to its strong taste, if you've never used ginger in a smoothie, start out with a small serving, and then increase as your taste buds allow! Ginger is great for cutting the green taste that comes with certain leafy greens.

It can be paired with berries, banana, and will do well with any leafy green. Try adding some ground or fresh ginger, but only a tiny pinch of each. This warming root is powerful, and a little goes a long way!

CINNAMON

Cinnamon is a great immune booster and contains both calcium and iron. Its warming scent is known to have a very energizing effect on the mind.

This spice is an excellent beverage enhancer, as it aids in the management of blood sugar and cholesterol levels. Cinnamon contains cinnamic acid, an antioxidant that helps to keep essential omega-3 fatty acids from oxidizing. Freshly grated or ground cinnamon are also good options.

Cinnamon is extremely high in antioxidants. This spice is also a potent anti-inflammatory, and there have been numerous studies showing the benefits of daily cinnamon consumption and the treatment of chronic issues like arthritis and certain autoimmune disorders.

Regular consumption of cinnamon has been linked to lowered blood glucose. However, one of the best benefits of daily consumption of cinnamon is that it's been scientifically proven to be a natural anti-cancer agent.

Cinnamon is spicy and slightly sweet which give smoothies a pleasant and distinct flavor. Cinnamon works best in creamier smoothies, and with ingredients like banana, oats and apples.

TURMERIC

Known as the King of all Spices for its potential role in natural healing as it's actually been proven to ease arthritis pain and could help prevent Alzheimer's disease. It can be used when you need to ease aches and decrease inflammation.

Turmeric is an Indian root that looks a bit like ginger. Known for its antioxidant properties, it promotes the healthy metabolism of fats and carbohydrates and may offer benefits to sufferers of digestive and inflammatory issues.

Peel and grate turmeric to blend into a variety of beverages. Its appetizing flavor is great in green smoothies that include carrot or pineapple.

Turmeric contains the powerful compound curcumin, which helps with inflammation, aids in digestion, fights cancer, eases arthritis, and lowers the risk of heart attacks. Turmeric has been shown to help protect the brain and it helps keep the brain functioning at its best and brightest. Adaptogens like turmeric help your body naturally acclimate to changing environments. Adaptogens have evolved over thousands of years to support and improve the body's ability to stay in balance and function optimally during times of stress.

Another way that turmeric can be useful is in easing joint pain, muscle fatigue and even arthritis. Turmeric is mildly aromatic and has hints of orange or ginger. It has a pungent, bitter flavor. Turmeric's strong flavor is best complemented by creamier fruits like banana or mango.

NUTMEG
Nutmeg contains fiber, manganese, thiamin, vitamin B6, folate, magnesium, and copper. Nutmeg has been known to possibly relieve pain, soothe indigestion, and strengthen cognitive function.

Nutmeg has a distinct, earthy flavor. You can pair it with cinnamon and apple to create a warming and spicy smoothie.

CAYENNE PEPPER
Cayenne is rich in multiple vitamins and minerals including vitamin C, vitamin B6, vitamin E, potassium, manganese, and flavonoids. It's because of these nutrients that cayenne has been proven to ease an upset stomach, ulcers, sore throats, irritating coughs, and diarrhea. Cayenne is also a well-known digestive aid. It stimulates the digestive tract, increasing the flow of enzyme production and gastric juices. This boosts metabolism and can help the body get rid of toxins.

Try cayenne with sweeter fruits like pineapple or mango.

Ground red pepper adds a spicy kick to your green smoothie, so use it sparingly. It also boosts your circulation, speeds up your metabolism, and curbs your appetite.

BASIL
Basil isn't just for pesto or Italian sauce. This herb is a little sweet and a little spicy, with notes of anise, mint and cloves. Like cilantro, basil is also known for its antibacterial properties and for helping with kidney

detoxification. Basil has a warm flavor that will boost your green smoothies and strengthen your kidneys. The kidneys play a major role in removing waste products and toxins from your bloodstream, like those produced from a diet that includes highly processed foods.

CHAPTER 4

AFTER THE PROGRAM

AFTER THE 12 DAY POWER DETOX PROGRAM

You can continue to enjoy the green smoothies either as breakfast and/or dinner meal while making healthy meal choices after the 12 Day Power Detox Program. You'll transition into eating healthier by using the tips in this book or you can start working with Health & Fitness Coach Ade to achieve your health and fitness goals via one of her online programs.

Visit **www.itstimefitnessaz.com/discovery-session** to schedule a complimentary Discovery Session.

If your goal is to continue to lose weight after the 12 Day Power Detox Program, note that healthy weight loss is about 1 to 2 pounds per week even though you may have experienced more weight loss during the 12 Day Power Detox Program.

SAMPLE HEALTHY EATING RECIPES

Lettuce Wrap
The idea is to substitute a sandwich bun for lettuce. On a regular healthy meal plan, the filling can be seasoned ground chicken, a variety of vegetables and spices. This can be used for the lunch on Day 11, Day 12 and The Modified Detox Program (without meat and cheese).

Veggie Medley Chopped Salad
This can be used for the lunch on Day 11, Day 12 and The Modified Detox Program. Combine cooked quinoa, carrot, bell pepper, cucumber, cherry tomatoes, corn (fresh or frozen) and pumpkin seeds (or any nuts) in a salad bowl. To make the dressing, mix garlic powder, ginger, salt, paprika, dried oregano, cayenne pepper and 1 tablespoon of olive oil in a small bowl then drizzle on the salad and enjoy.

Nutty Fruit Vegetable Salad:
This can be used for the lunch on Day 11, Day 12 and The Modified Detox Program. Put a blend of romaine lettuce, cucumber, carrot and red cabbage, 5 strawberries (sliced), toasted pecans or almonds in a salad bowl. To make the dressing, mix a 1 tablespoon of citrus juice, salt, black pepper, dried oregano, and 1 tablespoon of olive oil in a small bowl then drizzle on the salad and enjoy.

Southwest Chopped Salad

Put chopped green cabbage and romaine lettuce, along with carrots, radishes, cilantro and green onions in a salad bowl. Add roasted pumpkin seeds for a crunchy taste. Combine black beans, bell peppers, red onion, cilantro, in a bowl and toss on the salad. To make the dressing, mix garlic powder, ginger, salt, paprika, dried oregano, cayenne pepper and 1 tablespoon of olive oil in a small bowl then drizzle on the salad and enjoy.

Vegetable Soup

This can be used for the lunch on Day 11, Day 12 and The Modified Detox Program. Warm up water in the saucepan; add chopped green and red cabbage, broccoli, carrot, red bell pepper, jicama and green onions. Add more water if needed to cover the vegetables. Season with your favorite herbs and spices or use a mix of garlic powder, ginger, salt, paprika, dried oregano, cayenne pepper and 1 tablespoon of olive oil. Cook until the flavors come together and the vegetables and greens are tender, about 15 minutes or more. Serve hot, and garnish as desired.

Hot Oatmeal with unsweetened Raisins and unsweetened Almond Milk

This is one of my favorite go-to breakfast meals. Oatmeal is high in fiber so this keeps your stomach filled thereby avoiding early morning cravings. Add 1 cup of oats and a pinch of salt to boiling water and then let it simmer for a few minutes, stirring occasionally until thickened. Turn off the heat, stir in unsweetened raisins, a spoonful of sliced almonds and add unsweetened almond milk. I like the unsweetened vanilla almond milk.

Oat-Quinoa Fufu with Vegetable Stew

Fufu, also known as *okele*, is a popular African dish made from different types of flour. The flour used for the fufu in this recipe is a blend of oat and quinoa flour. Slowly pour 2/3 cup of flour blend into a small pot of boiling water. Stir constantly until the mixture thickens. Serve with a vegetable stew of your choice. You could try Spinach or Collard Greens cooked in a rich tomato sauce. You can also switch the fufu with 1 cup of cooked brown rice to make another yummy meal.

On a regular healthy meal plan, you could add meat i.e. grilled chicken or fish to the salad, soup and stew to give them a protein boost.

CHAPTER 5

12 DAY POWER DETOX DEVOTIONAL

INTRODUCTION

This 12-day devotional will guide you through the process of rejuvenating your soul and spirit by detoxing negative emotions while embracing positive emotions.

As you may know, man is a three-part being comprised of a spirit, soul and body. Your soul is the dimension of man which deals with the mental realm. It consists of the mind, will and emotions. It's the part that reasons, speaks and feels.

Emotions are the responses or feelings we have to the information coming to us from the physical world around us and from our perceptions or thoughts about what is taking place around us. We respond to emotions by crying, laughing, making facial expressions etc.

Our emotions tell us something about ourselves and a situation. They send us a message which could be good or bad. How we respond to the message we perceive, ultimately is what makes the difference.

The soul not only keeps a memory of things which have happened in our lives but the way we felt about those things. Everybody wants to feel happy, loved, confident, inspired, cheerful, grateful and accepted.

We feel different emotions throughout the day. If an emotion lasts longer than a few seconds, it could turn into a mood. It is important to understand the way we feel so that we can address it as soon as we are in the right frame of mind to do so.

When we experience negative emotions, the way we handle them depends on how healed or whole we are. This negative experience will either take you to the healed or unhealed zone. If you're in the healed zone, you will be better prepared to respond instead of reacting to the situation.

If you are not completely healed yet, it takes you to a place in the past where you had a similar experience, because your soul has memory and you may begin to react from that experience.

If you have a physical wound, and it is not properly treated, it could turn into an infection. At this point, you would not merely put a bandage over the wound, you would have to clean the wound, apply an ointment then put a bandage over it. The same applies to situations where our soul gets wounded. You need to take that mask off, expose it to the light, and apply the healing and germ-killing light of Christ into that wound so that it can heal.

Think about an unpleasant situation that keeps happening repeatedly, who is the common denominator in all these scenarios? Ouch!

This is why it is important to take time to heal your soul.

In this book, there are twelve devotions that coincide with each day of the 12 Day Power Detox Program. The devotion will address a common negative emotion people experience. To get the most out of your devotion time, you need to reflect, let the Holy Spirit reveal, then release the negative emotion and allow God to restore your soul. Soul healing is a continuous process as long as we live. As we periodically detox our bodies, we should also take time again to detox our souls.

Say this Bible verse as a prayer to begin this journey of detoxing your soul;

> Search me [thoroughly], O God, and know my heart; Test me and know my anxious thoughts; And see if there is any wicked or hurtful way in me, And lead me in the everlasting way." **Psalm 139:23-24, AMP**

THE EMOTIONAL DETOX PROCESS

Each day as you read your devotion, you will go through a series of steps to address a negative emotion. Spend time throughout the day to *reflect, reveal, release, restore, and pay attention* to how you are responding to negative situations.

As you go through each step, ask the Holy Spirit to show you any extra step(s) to take. Write down your "aha" moments, takeaways and lessons in a journal so that you don't forget. Better still; share it with a friend or in our Private Facebook Support Group.

STEP 1 - REFLECT

Reflecting allows you to thoughtfully look at past experiences once again, and learn how it affects your disposition towards life and different scenarios you find yourself in.

The first step is to identify the negative emotion and define it. Consider the following:

- Areas of your life and people you've attached to this negative emotion.

- Experiences from the past that are keeping you attached to this emotion.

- Triggers; something that brings back the memory of a negative incident or experience. A person's triggers can be activated through one or more of the five senses; sight, sound,   touch, smell and taste.

Find a quiet place and think carefully. Give yourself enough time to recall information from the past, then write down your reflections in a journal.

STEP 2 - REVEAL

The process of writing down your reflections in Step 1 is revealing. As you express your thoughts in writing, something is revealed. The revelation brings your thoughts and experiences into the present so that God can heal you.

Negative Emotions

Each time you feel a negative emotion, ask yourself questions to examine what's going on in your soul. Have you hidden your emotions from people? It's time to uncover it. Why am I feeling this way? How does this experience make me feel?

Attitude

Check your attitude. Attitudes are connected to emotions or experiences. Do you have a positive or negative attitude towards it? Have you really resolved the issue attached to the negative emotions? If someone was involved and the person walked into the room right now, will the first thought in your mind be positive or negative?

Your Part

What part did you have to play in the addressed situation? Did someone tell you they were offended by what you did? Please keep in mind that this process should never be done in a way to produce self-condemnation.

Examine how you communicate with people. Do you communicate how you are feeling or do you expect people to read your mind? Not communicating your thoughts could lead to misunderstanding and offense.

Recognize the Enemy's Strategy

Reveal the enemy's strategy in the situation. The goal of the enemy is to steal, kill and destroy (John 10:10). He wants to get us filled up and weighed down with emotional baggage inside and negative feelings in our hearts against one another, ourselves, and God. To keep him from getting the advantage over us, we should be familiar with his schemes, tactics and intentions (2 Corinthians 2:11; 1 Peter 5:8). He wants us to believe lies that do not line up with the truth of the Bible.

Allow the Holy Spirit to Search Your Heart

Finally, ask the Holy Spirit to search your heart to reveal anything not uncovered (Psalm 139:23–24). He will reveal to you anyone you may be holding a grudge against in your heart due to unforgiveness, hurt, pain, discord, etc.

STEP 3 - RELEASE

The next step is release. What experiences or thoughts related to the negative emotion have you held onto? It's time to let go of the hurt and pain. It's time to forgive and free yourself of the burden of negative emotions.

To release, you must be ready to own your mistakes, identify your triggers, and ready to forgive yourself and others so your heart can begin to heal. This is the only way you can truly get the full benefit of this process. You must be willing to let go of everything associated with the negative emotion.

Release anyone involved including you by saying a prayer of blessing over them. This should be a seasonal exercise. Do this step as often as you need to. This step is important because when you let go, you make room to receive positive experiences and thoughts.

Your willingness to release makes the next step quicker to complete.

STEP 4 - RESTORE

Restoration is the process that brings you to the healed zone. Healing is not complete till restoration comes. You can be restored when you allow God to do the healing work in your heart. God is the restorer of souls (Psalm 23:3). He restores us by His Holy Spirit which lives inside of us as His children and cleanses us by the washing of water with His word (Ephesians 5:26). He created our souls and knows the state it needs to be to function properly.

During the 12 Day Power Detox Program, you will be drinking smoothies made with a variety of fresh green vegetables and fruits. You will also be feeding your soul and spirit with the fruit of the Spirit: love, joy, peace, patience, kindness, goodness, faithfulness, gentleness and self-control (Galatians 5:22–23).

Each negative emotion will be paired with a positive emotion or response. The goal is to practice the positive response from a healed place and as you meditate on the given scriptures. You empower what you focus on and this eventually becomes what you receive and who you become.

Each devotion has faith declarations that will realign you with the way God sees you. They are faith statements based on God's word. Since we know God's word is quick, powerful and produces intended results, we will base the declarations on it.

> *"For the word of God is quick, and powerful, and sharper than any two-edged sword, piercing even to the dividing asunder of soul and spirit, and of the joints and marrow, and is a discerner of the thoughts and intents of the heart."* Hebrews 4:12

When you have God's word in you, it makes it easier to hear from God in that area and to judge your thoughts and actions by His Word. Be open to letting God speak to you through His Word.

I encourage you to say the declarations in front of a mirror. A mirror reflects the image it sees. The analogy is that you are observing yourself from the mirror of God's Word. God's Word gives you the desired image of who you are so the image you see right now may not be a physical representation of who God says you are. By saying the declarations based on

God's word, you are creating the image. As you say the declarations, begin to visualize the image of who you are becoming by faith, viewing yourself from the mirror of God's Word.

Research has shown that you believe what you hear yourself say more than what you hear other people say. And replacing negative words with positive words has the potential to change perspectives, attitudes, and reactions regarding yourself, others and the circumstances in which we find ourselves. You must replace it with positive affirmations at least thirteen times before it begins to resonate with you.

I encourage you to keep the declarations as part of your daily routine till you see every word come to pass in your life. It takes thirty days to develop discipline, sixty days to form a habit, ninety days adapt a lifestyle. Say the declarations at least once a day; A good rule of thumb is to repeat the declarations for at least five minutes, three times each day–morning, mid-day and evening. You can also do it as many times you want in a single day. The more you hear them, the quicker they will transform your thinking.

Since the words you speak create pictures in your mind, these pictures become what we see and eventually believe. To experience the intended result, don't read the declarations but say the declarations aloud to yourself daily, with power, attention, strong desire, faith and persistence. You will begin to use your words to restore your soul to the healthy zone. You will create a new healthy lifestyle, total outlook and mindset. Restoration is a continuous process until the healing of your soul is complete, so don't give up.

STEP 5 - RESPONSE
This is how you will handle negative emotions if you experienced them again. How do you want to show up or respond as you experience negative emotions?

Remember, responding from a healed place is always the goal and not reacting from an unhealed place. If you think about the negative emotion addressed and you say, "I don't have a problem with this emotion," prepare a response if you ever encounter it in the future so that you are not caught unaware. Think about what your immediate response would be before you decide the next step of action. Take a deep breath or several, do something positively unusual like laughing or give a positive compliment as it applies to the situation.

Day 1

<u>CREATE IN ME A CLEAN HEART</u>

Create in me a clean heart, O God, and renew a right,
persevering, and steadfast spirit within me.
Psalm 51:10, AMPC

Therefore, since we have these [great and wonderful] promises,
beloved, let us cleanse ourselves from everything that contaminates
body and spirit, completing holiness [living a consecrated
life—a life set apart for God's purpose] in the fear of God.
2 Corinthians 7:1, AMP

Today's Bible verse, Psalm 51:10 should be a constant prayer in our lives. Spend today examining and positioning yourself for the next twelve days as you get rid of all uncleanness like bad habits, addictions, idols and any ungodly character. In a humble spirit receive and welcome the Word of God into your heart where it can be implanted and rooted as it contains the power to save your soul (James 1:21).

Bad habits, addictions and idols are things in your life that you consciously or unconsciously consider more important than God. An individual may have a habit or be addicted to almost anything like drinking alcohol, doing drugs, stealing, lying, overeating, shopping, and even compulsive cleaning. A good thing could also gradually become a bad habit, addiction or an idol if care is not taken to give more focus to God.

Ask yourself if you're ready to deal with "stuff" over the next twelve days. You may have to deal with situations from the past, an issue you thought was already resolved and a new situation testing your character.

The Bible says in 1 Corinthians 10:13 that the temptations in your life are no different from what others experience. And God is faithful and compassionate; you can trust Him to not let you be tempted, tried and tested beyond your ability and strength of resistance and power to endure. He will not allow the temptation to be more than you can stand. When you are tempted, He will show you a way out so that you can endure. He'll always be there to help you come through it so that you are capable, strong and powerful to endure it.

Take time to read through, understand and get familiar with the **Emotional Detox Process** on page 57. It will help you complete the steps below. Write down your "aha" moments, takeaways, answers and lessons learned in a journal so that you don't forget.

THE EMOTIONAL DETOX PROCESS

Reflect: What does uncleanliness mean to you? Identify bad habits, addictions, idols you struggle with and anything that contaminates the spirit, soul and body.

Reveal: Write down the answers that were revealed in your reflections.

Reveal the enemy's strategy in the situation (John 10:10). Did you lose your identity, hope, faith, trust in God, sense of purpose and direction, confidence, integrity, friendship, fellowship, etc.?

Release: What bad habits, addictions, idols and perpetual sin do you need to let go of?

Restore: Say the declarations below aloud to yourself with attention, power, strong desire, faith and persistence.

- *I declare that I am born of God. I live by the dictates of the Spirit of God, not by my flesh.*

- *I am the righteousness of God in Christ Jesus. I have dominion over my sinful nature.*

- *Jesus has set me free, so I am free from any bad habits, addictions and my sinful nature.*

- *I let go of all my idols and I choose to put God first in all things.*

- *I embrace holiness, living a consecrated life—a life set apart for*

God's purpose and in the fear of God in Jesus Name. Amen!

Response: If you are faced with a situation involving a habit, addiction or an idol you've identified, how will you respond? Write down your response in your detox journal.

Day 2

LET GO, LET GOD – UNFORGIVENESS

*Bearing graciously with one another, and willingly forgiving each
other if one has a cause for complaint against another;
just as the Lord has forgiven you, so should you forgive.*
Colossians 3:13, AMP

Today we will deal with unforgiveness as it relates to actions and words.

Forgiveness is one of the first gifts we receive as children of God. It takes a willing heart to freely give the grace which we also have received from God. We were forgiven of our sins and the relationship with our heavenly Father was restored when we received His gift of forgiveness (1 John 1:9).

As God has forgiven us, He also expects us to forgive others. God takes forgiveness seriously and we see throughout the Bible that it is mentioned repeatedly.

Matthew 18:35 says God will deal with everyone who doesn't freely forgive others' offenses from the heart. Mark 11:25 also says that when we come before God in prayer, we should forgive anything we may have against anyone so that our Father in heaven will forgive the wrongs we have done.

How often should we forgive? Jesus said in Matthew 18:22 that we should forgive seventy times seven. Based on previous Bible verses, I would say as often as you need to.

Keep and guard your heart, for out of it flow the springs of life (Proverbs 4:23). The hardness of heart is one of the hindrances to forgiveness. People with hard hearts refuse to forgive or humble themselves to ask for forgiveness. They say I forgive you, but never let go. They ask for forgiveness then go back to do the same thing again. The Bible says they are darkened in their understanding and separated from the life of God because of their ignorance and hardness of heart (Ephesians 4:18). Unforgiveness is one of Satan's most used weapons to gain a legal right to have access to our lives. It opens the door to satanic oppression, influence, sicknesses, diseases and the like. We need to get rid of offense before it leads to unforgiveness. If we don't, our unforgiveness can lead to anger, bitterness, violence, and hatred, which are some of the leading causes of crime in the world today.

You might say their words and actions towards you were mean leaving you in pain and hurt. This situation makes you vulnerable. Your flesh wants to take revenge, wishes something evil happens to them. However, the right thing to do is to let God handle it. Leave room for God to bring appropriate judgment.

> Beloved, never avenge yourselves, but leave the way open for God's wrath [and His judicial righteousness]; for it is written [in Scripture], "Vengeance is Mine, I will repay," says the Lord. **Romans 12:19 AMP**

Take time to read through, understand and get familiar with the **Emotional Detox Process** on page 57. It will help you complete the steps below. Write down your "aha" moments, takeaways, answers and lessons learned in a journal so that you don't forget.

THE EMOTIONAL DETOX PROCESS

Reflect: Pray Psalm 139:23–24, AMP. Identify the areas where you have been offended in the past and who was involved as it comes to memory.

Reveal: Write down the answers revealed in your reflections. It could be the names of the people, an entity or organization. Sometimes we are upset with God because of unfulfilled expectations, or an incident you feel He could have prevented. As you yield to the Holy Spirit and ask Him to search your heart, you'll be surprised by the stuff He brings up.

Unforgiveness is like venom. It spreads when people start reacting because they are offended. Here's how to test if you've been hurt by someone or have unforgiveness in your heart. When you hear the person's name or see or communicate with them, you will have a negative reaction. You are not smiling, there may even be a frown on your face. When they communicate with you and show you love, it takes you a minute or even a while to walk in love towards them, so that you can receive their kind gesture.

When you are asked to do something for the person, there is hesitation even though it is in your power to do it.

What part did you have to play? Has someone told you they were offended by what you did?

Release: Release the people who have offended you. Say I let you go.

I release (Insert Name) from every unforgiveness (mention specific words or actions done to you, if you remember), I have against you. Breathe in and out as you speak these phrases. Releasing the baggage and burden of unforgiveness results in emotional weight loss, as well as physical weight loss in some cases.

Forgive yourself, let go of any unforgiveness you have against God. Break every evil and inappropriate thought processes and patterns that are self-sabotaging and self-defeating. Cast down every imagination and every high thing that exalts itself against the knowledge of God, bringing every negative thought into captivity to the obedience of Christ (2 Corinthians 10:5). We are going to replace that unforgiveness with agape, the unconditional love of God which is also a fruit of the Spirit.

Restore: Say the declarations below aloud to yourself with attention, power, strong desire, faith and persistence. Repeat it as many times as you need to until you see change happen.

- *The love of God is shed abroad in my heart by the Holy Spirit (Romans 5:5). I am a love being. I love people unconditionally just as Jesus loves me.*

- *I have the mind of Christ and hold the thoughts (feelings and purposes) of His heart (1 Corinthians 2:16). I love with the love of God, so I release you and forgive you (insert names of people, entities and yourself).*

- *I forgive you for your hurtful words and actions towards me, and the pain you caused me as a result.*

- *"As God's own chosen one, I am set apart and sanctified for His purpose. I am dearly loved by God Himself, I put on a heart of compassion, kindness, humility, gentleness, and patience and I receive the power to endure whatever injustice or unpleasantness comes, with a good temper." (Colossians 3:12)*

- *I strive to live in peace with everybody and pursue that consecration and holiness (Hebrews 12:14). In Jesus Name. Amen!*

Response: If you are faced with a situation where you must forgive the same person or entity that hurt you in the past, how will you respond?

Write down your response in your detox journal. Ask God for wisdom (James 1:5). Seek godly counsel from a trusted person who will not take sides. Every time you relive a similar experience to what you've had in the past, there is an emotion attached to it, the emotion could be positive or negative. How you respond or react to it will determine if you have been totally healed from that experience.

Be humble. Apologize when you realize you hurt someone's feelings or treated someone unfairly. Make sure you really mean it because people can tell when you are sincere. You can go a step further by asking them how you can prevent a similar dispute from happening in the future. This step takes a lot of humility.

Day 3

LET IT GO – UNFORGIVENESS

Let all bitterness and indignation and wrath (passion, rage, bad temper) and resentment (anger, animosity) and quarreling (brawling, clamor, contention) and slander (evil-speaking, abusive or blasphemous language) be banished from you, with all malice (spite, ill will, or baseness of any kind). And become useful and helpful and kind to one another, tenderhearted (compassionate, understanding, loving-hearted), forgiving one another [readily and freely], as God in Christ forgave you.
Ephesians 4:31–32, AMPC

Above all things have intense and unfailing love for one another, for love covers a multitude of sins [forgives and disregards the offenses of others].
1 Peter 4:8, AMPC

We are spending more time on unforgiveness because it is one of the ways the enemy brings oppression and sickness in the lives of the children of God. Today we will be dealing with unforgiveness as it relates to emotions; how we feel.

People will always remember how you made them feel. The soul not only keeps a memory of things which have happened in our lives but the way we felt about those things. As long as you deal with people in your daily life, your feelings will get hurt from time to time.

Every pain and hurt you feel is valid. How you heal from the negative experience is what makes a difference.

Hurting people react based on feelings. They rehearse in their minds how they are going to prove that they were right and the other person was wrong. When they allow their flesh to rule them, they practice what they will say when they confront the person who hurt them.

Marianne Williamson once said, "*Unforgiveness is like drinking poison and waiting for the other person to die.*" It can affect your physical health, mental health and spiritual well-being. It can affect how we relate with people, even the people not involved in the offense.

Forgiving means giving in advance when it's not deserved; fore give. We must forgive others so that we can be forgiven by God (Matthew 6:14–15).

Forgiveness is not a feeling, it is a choice and an act of compassion to release the desire to punish someone or yourself for an offense. As you have received grace, you can give grace too. Forgiveness is not a hard thing, but must always come from your heart.

Forgiving doesn't mean forgetting or ignoring hurtful actions done and words said to us. We should not pretend like it never happened. Forgiveness doesn't mean you have to be friends with the person or put yourself in an abusive or harmful situation.

Forgiveness is deciding that the people who offended you no longer owe you anything, including an apology or even acknowledging the hurt. Forgiveness allows you to shift your focus from the pain to God. It allows more room in your life for Him; His plan and purpose, His love, joy and peace.

Even though you are the one who feels the hurt and pain carrying the burden, the other person may be out there having a good time. You only have control over what happens to you, so making the choice to start the healing process is up to you.

Take time to read through, understand and get familiar with the **Emotional Detox Process** on page 57. It will help you complete the steps below. Write down your "aha" moments, takeaways, answers and lessons in a journal so that you don't forget.

THE EMOTIONAL DETOX PROCESS

Reflect: On Day 2, you identified the areas where you have been offended in the past and who was involved. Now identify the feelings, such as negative emotions you felt when those actions were done and words were said to you.
Reveal: Write down how the experience made you feel. Did you feel

unwelcomed, rejected, betrayed, unimportant, desperate, not good enough etc.?

Examine how you communicate with people. Do you communicate how you are feeling or do you expect people to read your mind? Not communicating your thoughts could lead to misunderstanding and offense. Don't make assumptions that they know, you may be wrong.

Consider the enemy's strategy in the situation identified (John 10:10). Did you lose your joy, peace, trust, friendship, hope, patience, integrity, etc.?

Put your expectations in God. Commit your plans to Him and trust them wholly to Him; He will cause your thoughts to become agreeable to His will, and so shall your plans be established and succeed (Proverbs 16:3). When you need help, first ask God who you should reach out to, that way you can ask the right person.

Release: Release the people who have offended you based on how they made you feel.

- *I choose to forgive (insert name). I forgive (insert name) for their action and words towards me which made me feel (name the negative feelings still in your heart). I repent and renounce all the lies (state the lies) I believed about (insert name) and the judgment against (insert name). Lord, I am choosing to let go, not hold it against them anymore or seek revenge. I release (name) into your hands.*

- *Dear God, I ask that you forgive me for holding unforgiveness in my heart against them for this long. I break off any soul ties of unforgiveness and its consequence between me and (insert name).*

- *Jesus, I receive your freedom. I am free from any torment, guilt, bondage or condemnation. I close every open door to Satan in my life and I receive the complete healing of my soul in Jesus Name. Amen!*

- *Forgiveness brings freedom. If you are having a hard time releasing someone, you may need to spend more time to study and meditate on the Bible verses addressing unforgiveness.*

Restore: Say the prayer of faith below with a heart of repentance.

Dear God, I ask that you bless (insert name). I pray that (insert name) will prosper and be in good health even as his/her soul prospers. I bless the works of his/her hands. Help me to be kind, tenderhearted, understanding and loving-hearted towards (insert name) In Jesus Name. Amen!

Response: If you experience a situation where your feelings are hurt, what will be your immediate response? How you respond or react to it will determine if you have been totally healed from an experience. Write down your response in your detox journal.

Day 4

DEALING WITH OVERWHELMING FEELINGS

Come to Me, all you who labor and are heavy-laden and overburdened and I will cause you to rest. [I will ease and relieve and refresh your souls.] Take My yoke upon you and learn of Me, for I am gentle (meek) and humble (lowly) in heart, and you will find rest (relief and ease and refreshment and [recreation and blessed quiet) for your souls. For My yoke is wholesome (useful, good—not harsh, hard, sharp, or pressing, but comfortable, gracious, and pleasant), and My burden is light and easy to be borne. **Matthew 11:28–30, AMPC**

Today we will address the emotions that overwhelm; fear, anxiety, stress and worry.

Being overwhelmed emotionally may be caused by stress at home or work, traumatic life experiences, relationship issues, and much more. Your emotions can be intense and last from a few hours to as long as a few days depending on how you address them.

A person is most likely to be overwhelmed by negative emotions, such as extreme sadness, persistent anger, fear, anxiety, or guilt. A person who is emotionally overwhelmed may become irritable or depressed, experience significant anxiety and panic, stress over things that may be of little significance, or have an inability to distinguish thoughts or beliefs from reality. Overwhelming emotions can lead to self-destructive behaviors such as substance abuse or self-injury.

Short-term effects of stress include headaches, shallow breathing, difficulty sleeping, anxiety, and upset stomach. Long-term chronic stress can increase the risk of heart disease, back pain, depression, persistent muscle aches and pains, and a weakened immune system.

When you're in a high-pressure situation, examine your train of thought to see if it's adding to the stress you feel.

Perhaps, you felt overworked, scared, and stressed with a project you were required to finish at work. Then, when you went home, you suddenly felt pressured by your kids or your spouse to have something that needs your immediate attention. There is just so much to do. But, if you think back, it started with the project at work.

It's not the project at work and the series of events after that created stress. It's the way a person responds to the different situations like urgencies and demands of work, financial problems, relationship meltdowns, etc. that make them feel stressed. If you respond to added stress by eating more, you could end up with added pounds. Emotional eating may be caused by different triggers in men and women. Know your triggers. No one can avoid all stress but it's always best to keep unhealthy levels in check when possible.

God constantly reassures us in His Word that He is with us; He will not leave us or abandon us (Hebrews 13:5). He is for us and nothing can stand against us (Romans 8:31).

The Bible says in 1 John 4:18 that *"there is no fear in love. Dread does not exist, but full-grown and perfect love turns fear out of the door and expels every trace of terror. Fear brings with it the thought of punishment, and whoever is afraid has not reached the full maturity of love [is not yet grown into love's complete perfection]."*

I have found that to deal with fear, you must face the fear. Procrastination doesn't make it go away. Doing it afraid is being courageous. Finding confidence and credibility in yourself or in what you do really helps. Then you will begin to find out that *"F. E. A. R."* is only *False Evidence Appearing Real. God has not given you the Spirit of fear but of love, power and a sound mind* (2 Timothy 1:7).

Worry is like a spinning wheel that never stops. When worry is internalized, it can turn into depression. Instead of worrying the Bible says do not worry about your life, what you will eat or drink; or about your body, what you will wear (Matthew 6:25). Don't worry about tomorrow; let it take care of itself. Focus on each day's trouble and handle them one at a time. Also know that God knows what you need and He will provide your needs when you ask Him.

Take time to read through, understand and get familiar with the **Emotional**

Detox Process on page 57. It will help you complete the steps below. Write down your "aha" moments, takeaways, answers and lessons in a journal so that you don't forget.

THE EMOTIONAL DETOX PROCESS

Reflect: Identify how you react to overwhelming feelings like fear, anxiety, stress and worry. Common effects include sleep problems, skin rashes, fatigue, irritability, agitation, headache, depression, excessive worrying, mood swings, chest pain, anxiety, upset stomach, ulcers, and high blood pressure.

When are you most vulnerable to the overwhelming feelings? Prepare yourself for those moments.

Why do you feel overwhelmed? Whenever you're feeling overwhelmed, simply ask yourself where the feelings are coming from. Are they stemming from one incident? If they are, then it's easier to detach from your feelings of being overwhelmed. You know what's causing it. The simple act of being aware of why you are feeling overwhelmed can be enough to free yourself from repeating the same thing in other areas of your life.

Reveal: Write down the answers revealed by your reflections and the questions below.

- When did the overwhelmed feeling start? Did it all start with one event? Identify the one thing that makes you feel overwhelmed. Is it fear, anxiety, stress or worry?

- Are you most affected at a particular time of the day, week, month or year? Be specific. Is it in the morning, on Mondays or in the Winter?

- Are you allowing your imagination to run wild, over-exaggerating the situation before it happens or thinking the worst or making it a far worse outcome than is likely?

- Why do you feel the way you feel? Where is the overwhelming feeling coming from? Trace it back to the original incident that started the feeling.

- What types of situations make you feel overwhelmed? What were your thoughts really consumed with when you were completely overwhelmed?

- Is the situation likely to affect other aspects of your life? Are you promising to do more than you can handle?

- Do you procrastinate, and then you end up completing a task under pressure?

- Are you triggered to eat from stress as a way to deal with difficult emotions?

Release: Release the overwhelming feelings of fear, anxiety, stress and worry in a current situation that you're going through. As you read, pray and declare these verses.

Dear God, I come to You to release the weight and burden of (insert the overwhelming feelings). Forgive me for not trusting You completely with every area of my life. I cast all my cares on you, God, knowing that you will provide all that I need. You sustain me (Psalm 55:22).

As I wait on You Lord, renew me with Your strength and power so that I do not become weak, tired, and anxious (Isaiah 40:31).

Help me to no longer be agitated, disturbed, fearful, intimidated and unsettled about the situations I face in life (John 14:27).

Free me from the spirit of timidity (of cowardice, of craven and cringing and fawning fear), and fill me with the spirit of power, love and a calm and well-balanced mind and discipline and self-control (2 Timothy 1:7).

Strengthen my faith so that I am not moved by what I feel, my thoughts or situation. Let me be moved only by Your Word and promises. I will not be overwhelmed by (insert the overwhelming feelings) because You are with me. Lord, I receive the strength and help that comes from You. Thank You for upholding me with Your victorious right hand (Isaiah

41:10) in Jesus Name. Amen!

Restore: When you regain control over your thoughts, you can move forward with your life rather than continuing to get caught up in overwhelming emotions. You will no longer feel emotionally overwhelmed because you've gained a new understanding of yourself. You're once again in control of your thoughts and not the other way around.

Say the declarations below aloud to yourself with attention, power, strong desire, faith and persistence. Repeat it as many times as you need to until you see change happen.

- *I enter the rest of the Lord concerning (insert the overwhelming situation). I am confident and trust in the Lord with all my heart and mind. I do not rely on my own insight or understanding but in all my ways, I recognize and acknowledge Him, and He directs my paths **(Proverbs 3:5– 6).***

- *I do not fear or have any anxiety about anything, but in every circumstance and in everything, by prayer, I make my definite requests known to God, with thanksgiving. I received God's peace which transcends all understanding to know that God takes cares of all my needs **(Philippians 4:6–8)** in Jesus Name. Amen!*

Response: If you experience overwhelming feelings like fear, anxiety, stress and worry, how will you respond?

Here are some suggestions. Get organized by using a daily planner to write out and prioritize tasks. Get rid of distractions and focus one task at a time. Set limits; don't agree to unnecessary, stressful obligations. Get physically active and eat a healthy diet. Aim for eight hours of sleep each night.

Understand what stresses you. Both positive and negative situations can tip the scales in your life. On the negative side, financial difficulties, divorce, criticism by a friend or boss, unrealistic work demands, or death of a friend or family member can cause stress. On the positive side, getting married, being promoted, having a baby, moving to a new home—even going on vacation—can be stressful.

Respond to fear with faith believing in God that all things are working together and fitting into a plan for good because you love God and are called according to His design and purpose (Romans 8:28).

Wait patiently after you've prayed believing that the answer to your requests will be fulfilled and let the peace of God settle any doubts and questions in your mind.

Day 5

DEALING WITH JOY KILLERS

This [day in which God has saved me] is the day which the Lord has made; Let us rejoice and be glad in it. **Psalm 118:24, AMP**

The thief comes only in order to steal and kill and destroy. I came that they may have and enjoy life, and have it in abundance [to the full, till it overflows]. **John 10:10, AMP**

Each day presents the opportunity to forget the sorrows of yesterday and welcome the new day with joy (Psalm 30:5). Today we will deal with joy killers like anger, grief, sadness, depression and bitterness.

Jesus came so that you may enjoy life in abundance until it overflows into the lives of others. The abundant life includes a life filled with joy as we enjoy God's rich blessings.

The devil's plot is to first steal your joy, if he's given the opportunity, he will proceed to kill your joy and finally destroy it. This is why the Bible warns us not to give room to the devil so that he can lead us to sin. He is on a mission, roaming around, seeking who he can prey upon (1 Peter 5:8). We must be alert and aware of his schemes. Resist the devil, and he will flee from you (James 4:7).

Anger is an outward expression of a deeper emotion or feeling. It is fed by feelings of disappointment, hurt, frustration, rejection, and embarrassment.

People get upset when one of their values is compromised. When you don't process your pain, you can become angry. From this, we can discover that an angry man is someone who has not learned how to process his pain.

Let's face it, anger is an ugly emotion. James 1:20 says it does not promote the righteousness of God. Quick tempers can result in an outburst of emotions thereby hurting yourself and others. James 1:19 advises us to be quick to hear. Be a ready listener, slow to speak, slow to take offense and slow to get angry.

Bitterness is usually associated with anger and holding a grudge. When you are offended or disappointed by others and allow the hurt to grow in your heart, bitterness and resentment will take root. It's your duty to make sure that you don't fall short of the grace of God; that no root of bitterness springs up and causes trouble which makes many to be defiled (Hebrews 12:15).

Grief is a natural response to losing someone or something that's important to you who you have a bond with or affection for. You may feel a variety of emotions, like sadness or loneliness. To heal from grief, you must give yourself time. Accept your feelings and know that grieving is a process. Don't isolate yourself. Spend time with friends and family. Get back to the activities that bring you joy.

Depression is a mood disorder that causes a persistent feeling of sadness and loss of interest. The low mood lingers day-after-day, enough to interrupt daily activities. Difficult life situations can trigger depression, like losing a loved one, getting fired from a job, going through a divorce, etc. Activities that were once pleasurable lose their appeal. A depressed person experiences a sense of guilt, worthlessness or a lack of hope and can also experience serious weight loss or weight gain.

Job was a man mentioned in the Bible who went through a period of depression. He suffered great loss, devastation and physical illness but God restored all that he lost when he forgave his friends and prayed for them (Job 42:10). He blessed him with twice as much as he had before.

Happiness is based on what you have while joy is intangible. Joy is not an emotion but a fruit of the Holy Spirit. So, you have access to it, if you are filled with the Spirit of God. Happiness is what you have after you see it or while you have it in your life. It is tied to the tangible things we see. Joy is what you have while you're waiting for it and what you have when you receive it. You can be happy and joyful at the same time. Joy is tied to your faith, belief and hope in God Who specializes in the impossible. In essence, you do not need to see it to be joy-full. You may not always be able to maintain your happiness but strive to maintain your joy by staying in the presence of God. In his presence is fullness of joy (Psalm 16:11).

If you don't control the joy killers and you let them linger for too long, it gives the devil an opportunity to lead you into offense, revenge or any other kind of sin. You have yielded to the flesh and are no longer being led by the Holy Spirit (Ephesians 4:27). Your anger should not last long. The Bible tells us to get rid of anger before the sun goes down (Ephesians 4:26).

When you realize your own failures, how you reacted to what was done to you and you take responsibility for what you've allowed into your mind and life, then you can begin to heal your emotions. Blaming others will hinder the healing power of the Holy Spirit in our lives; therefore, it must be dealt with before healing can freely flow into our mind and emotions.

Take time to read through, understand and get familiar with the **Emotional Detox Process** on page 57. It will help you complete the steps below. Write down your "aha" moments, takeaways, answers and lessons in a journal so that you don't forget.

THE EMOTIONAL DETOX PROCESS

Reflect: Identify the areas where you were or are experiencing joy-killers like anger, grief, sadness, depression and bitterness in the past or in a current situation that you're going through. Who was involved as it comes to memory? How have or do you react? When are you most vulnerable? Now prepare yourself. Why do you feel anger, grief, sadness, depression and bitterness?

Reveal: Write down how the experience made you feel? Unwelcomed, rejected, betrayed, unimportant, desperate, not good enough, etc.?

Who was involved? Are you angry towards God, yourself, others or an entity? Do you keep blaming others for your emotions without owning up to your own mistakes?

What part did you have to play? Did someone tell you they were offended by what you did?

Release: Release the people or entities who have offended you based on how they made you feel. Ask God what you can do to be healed. Ask for wisdom.

Say out loud these declarations.

- *I choose to forgive (insert name or entity). I forgive (insert name or entity) for their action and words towards me which made me feel (name the negative feelings still in your heart).*

- *I repent and renounce all the lies (state the lies) I believed about (insert name or entity) and the judgment against (insert name or entity). Lord I am choosing to let go, not hold it against them anymore or seek revenge. I release (insert name or entity) into your hands.*

- *I let go of anger, grief, sadness, depression and bitterness and put it on the cross of Calvary where Jesus bore my grief, and carried my sorrows, pain, and affliction. By Your stripes, I am healed (Isaiah 53:4–5). I open my heart for healing to begin (Imagine you did this in front of the Cross). I receive Your love into my heart to love them as I love myself.*

- *Dear God, I ask that You forgive me for holding it against them this long. I break off any soul ties of unforgiveness and its consequence. Jesus, I receive Your freedom. I am free me from any torment, guilt, bondage or condemnation. I close every open door to Satan in my life and I receive the complete healing of my soul.*

With a blank piece of paper before you, ask God to bring to mind anyone you need to forgive. If he gives you a name or two or ten, start praying for those on your list. Pray every day until you feel God melt that resentment you've been holding onto. I have found it is impossible to be unforgiving toward those I am praying for. It's not easy to start praying for them; it's one of the hardest things I've done. But when I make that person an object of prayer, I open the door of my heart a little wider so that God can come in and breathe on my hardened heart, melting the icy resentment that is there.

Restore: Say the prayer of faith below with a heart of repentance. Repeat it as many times as you need to do it to see change happen.

Dear God, I ask that you bless (insert name or entity). I bless them too. I pray that they will prosper and be in good health even as their soul prospers. I bless the works of their hands in Jesus Name. Amen!

This is the day the Lord has made. I will rejoice and be glad in it.

As I stand here in Your presence (Psalm 16:11), I receive the fullness of joy. Joy! Joy! Joy!

I pray that You will fill me with all joy, hope and peace in believing [through the experience of your faith] and by the power of the Holy Spirit, I will abound and be overflowing (bubbling over) with hope and joy (Romans 15:13). The joy of the Lord gives me strength (Nehemiah 8:10).

He helps me, and my heart is filled with joy (Psalm 28:7).

And with my song, I will thank and praise You, Lord (Psalm 28:7).

I will rejoice in Your mercy and be glad in Your unfailing love, (Psalm 31:7). I strive to live in peace with everybody and pursue that consecration and holiness (Hebrews 12:14).

Response: If you experience a situation with one of the joy killers, what will be your immediate response? How you respond or react to it will determine if you have been totally healed from an experience. What is your natural response to a negative situation? Do you respond with bitterness or love?

Smile, even if you don't feel it. The act of smiling changes your body chemistry. You'll suddenly feel happier! Laughter is also a great emotional release! Laughter releases chemical endorphins to make you feel happy and relaxed. You've heard laughter is good medicine how about laughter is free medicine. There's a wellspring of laughter waiting to overflow out of you and it doesn't cost anything. Well ... maybe a sad moment.

So why don't you take a minute or two, take yourself down memory lane to a place where you laughed hard or somewhere that you've been that makes you happy. I hope you feel better now!
We should be joy-givers, hope-bringers and peace-makers to people in our lives and help them remember what real grace is and where lasting

help is found.

People have different ways of viewing the world. The more positive outlook is being optimistic while the reverse is considered pessimistic. Your worldview dictates how you deal with most situations and even what you expect from the world around you. For example, you may have an optimistic outlook on life, but feel pessimistic about your job.

A pessimistic outlook may struggle with expressing gratitude, appreciating others and the simple things in life. It often comes off as mean even though this may not be what was intended. It is realistic and not in a world of fantasy. It tends to see failure before success. It also tends to focus on the past and use those experiences to predict future events. Conversely, the optimistic outlook will always see the good in every situation. It will cheer you up and encourage you.

When responding, always express gratitude first. Complaining is very unattractive and can leave you even more upset if you don't get what you want. Negative emotions have energy that can be transferred. Be careful not to transfer negative emotions to others when you share negative experiences.

When you give thanks, you get more out of life and blessings will be given to you. Instead of complaining about an unpleasant situation, try giving constructive feedback.

When you communicate, always start with giving thanks before you look at the negative outlook on life or your current unpleasant situation. Start with one thing you are thankful for during the experience, and then state your displeasure in the most loving way possible so that your conversation will be gracious and attractive, and you will have the right response for everyone (Colossians 4:6).

Taking the time to do what you love is good for your physical and mental health and it will help keep that smile on your face.

Day 6

<u>DEALING WITH UNFULFILLED EXPECTATIONS</u>

For I know the thoughts and plans that I have for you, says the Lord, thoughts and plans for welfare and peace and not for evil, to give you hope in your final outcome. **Jeremiah 29:11, AMPC**

For surely there is a latter end [a future and a reward], and your hope and expectation shall not be cut off. **Proverbs 23:18, AMPC**

Today we will address *unfulfilled* expectations disappointment, discouragement and failure.

These are the emotions you feel when things don't work the way you expected, or the outcome didn't meet your intended expectation or you didn't meet the set goal. Regardless of the outcome, remember that God's plans for you are good just like Jeremiah 29:11 states above.

Disappointment is the feeling of sadness or displeasure caused by the nonfulfillment of your hopes or expectations.

Discouragement steals your courage, hope or confidence. It is the state of having lost your confidence or enthusiasm for something.

Failure is the state or condition of not meeting a desirable or intended objective. It is a state of inability to perform a normal function.

When you experience unfulfilled expectations, don't let your emotions keep you down for too long. You need to get back up. As soon as you're up on your feet, you can begin to take the steps of faith to believe you can succeed again. If you decide to stay down too long, you'll begin to settle for the things at the bottom. The things that will draw you far away from God.

You can choose to let a setback redefine your life negatively or positively. It is ok to cry for a moment but after that, wipe away your tears and get up. Learn from the experience and turn it into a positive experience by choosing to continue to live your best life. The way I see it is... a setback is a set up for a comeback.

You will have failed attempts or unmet goals no matter how well prepared you are. How you perceive the situation determines how quickly you will recover from it.

Mind you, I didn't say you will fail but I called it failed attempts. If you've ever been successful at anything, you will know that the failed attempt doesn't define who you are. There will be more opportunities to come for you to be successful in the future.

Think about how a baby is conceived. There are usually so many failed attempts when sperm is trying to fertilize one egg. Do you think the mighty Creator of the heavens and earth couldn't have made this possible at one attempt? Absolutely, He could have but He allowed it, so we can learn a valuable lesson from the start. You were the successful attempt! Never ever think you are a failure because you've had failed attempts at something.

The fact that you were born and are alive today signifies that you are successful. You may experience failed attempts in relationships, marriage, education, business, ministry, career, etc. Whatever the case may be, the moment you showed up on planet earth and there was the sound of a baby crying, you were announcing your victory. Saying I'm here, I made it successfully. As far as I'm concerned, that's a successful start. You can choose to live life with this mindset, reminding yourself that you were born a success.

Despite all these things, you are more than conquerors and gain a surpassing victory through Jesus Who loves you (Romans 8:37, AMP).

Thanks be to God, Who in Christ always leads you in triumph [as trophies of Christ's victory] and through you spreads and makes evident the fragrance of the knowledge of God everywhere (2 Corinthians 2:14, AMPC).

Take time to read through, understand and get familiar with the **Emotional Detox Process** on page 57. It will help you complete the steps below. Write down your "aha" moments, takeaways, answers and lessons in a journal so that you don't forget.

THE EMOTIONAL DETOX PROCESS

Reflect: Identify the areas in the past or in a current situation when you experienced unfulfilled expectations like disappointment, discouragement or failure. Who is/was involved as it comes to memory?

How did you react to unfulfilled expectations? When are you most vulnerable? Prepare yourself. What was the reason you felt disappointed, discouraged or like a failure?

Reveal: Write down how the experience(s) made you feel? Did you feel unwelcomed, rejected, betrayed, unimportant, desperate, not good enough, etc.?

Who was involved? Are you angry towards God, yourself, others or an entity? Do you keep blaming others for your emotions without owning up to your own mistakes?

What part did you have to play? Did someone tell you they were offended by what you did? Did you give in to self-pity?

Release: Release the people or entities who have offended you based on how they made you feel, including yourself.

Ask God what you can do on your own side to be healed. Ask God for wisdom.

- *I choose to forgive (insert name or entity). I forgive (insert name or entity) for their action and words towards me which made me feel (name the negative feelings still in your heart). I repent and renounce all the lies (state the lies) I believed about (insert name or entity) and the judgment against (insert name or entity). Lord, I am choosing to let go, not hold it against them anymore or seek revenge. I release (insert name or entity) into your hands.*

- *I let go the disappointment, discouragement and failure and put it on the cross of Calvary where Jesus bore our griefs, and carried our sorrows [grief, pain, and affliction]. By your stripes, I am healed.*

(Isaiah 53:4–5). (Imagine you did this in front of a cross).

- *I open my heart for healing to begin I receive your love into my heart to love (insert name or entity) as I love myself.*

- *Dear God, I ask that you forgive me for holding it against them this long. I break off any soul ties of unforgiveness and its consequence Jesus, I receive your freedom. I am free me from any torment, guilt,-bondageor condemnation. I close every open door to Satan in my life and I receive the complete healing of my soul.*

Restore: Say the prayer of faith below with a heart of repentance. Repeat it as many times as you need to do it to see changes happen.

Dear God, I ask that you bless (insert name or entity). I bless them too. I pray that they will prosper and be in good health even as their soul prospers. I bless the works of their hands In Jesus Name. Amen!

This is the day the Lord has made. I will rejoice and be glad in it.

As I stand here in your presence (Psalm 16:11), I receive the fullness of joy. Joy! Joy! Joy!

I pray that you will fill me with all joy, hope and peace in believing [through the experience my faith] and by the power of the Holy Spirit, I will abound and be overflowing (bubbling over) with hope and joy. (Romans 15:13). The joy of the Lord gives me strength (Nehemiah 8:10)

He helps me, and my heart is filled with joy. And with my song, I will thank and praise you, Lord (Psalm 28:7)

I will rejoice in your mercy and be glad in Your unfailing love, (Psalm 31:7). I strive to live in peace with everybody and pursue that consecration and holiness. (Hebrews 12:14) in Jesus Name. Amen!

I speak Amos 9:13 as a prophetic declaration over you.

> *"Things are going to happen so fast your head will swim,*
> *one thing fast on the heels of the other. You won't be able to keep up.*
> *Everything will be happening at once and everywhere you look,*
> *blessings!Blessings like wine pouring off the mountains and hills.*
> *God is making everything right again for you."*

Response: If you experience a situation with one of the addressed unfulfilled expectations, how will you respond?

Understand your natural response to a negative situation. How you respond or react to it will determine if you have been totally healed from a past experience.

The best way to quickly get over a negative feeling is replacing it with a positive feeling. What positive feeling are you replacing it with?

Smile, even if you don't feel it. The act of smiling makes you feel happier! Laughter is also a great emotional release!

So why don't you take a minute or two, take yourself down memory lane to a place where an expectation was fulfilled. Recall how happy you felt. Hope that makes you feel better, now make it a great day.

Have an optimistic outlook towards life or surround yourself with people who are joy-givers, hope- bringers and encourages. This could be a prayer support group, family members or friends.

Express gratitude first. Be thankful in all things, this is God's will for your life (1 Thessalonians 5:18). He continuously gives us reasons to be thankful. We may not be able to give God thanks for the difficult situation that we find ourselves in, but we can learn to look for things we can be thankful for in the midst of it. Start with the small things and watch the list grow as you yield to the Holy Spirit to help you remember the blessings you already have in your life.

Keep declaring God's Word over the situation and believe change is coming soon.

Examine how you communicate with people. Do you communicate how you are feeling or you expect people to read your mind? Not communicating your thoughts could lead to misunderstanding and offense. Don't make assumptions that they should know, you may be wrong.

Put your expectations in God. If you need help, first ask God who you should reach out to, that way you can ask the right person.

Taking the time to do what you love is really good for your physical and mental health and to keep that smile on your face.

Day 7

DEALING WITH ACCUSATIONS

Therefore, [there is] now no condemnation (no adjudging guilty of wrong) for those who are in Christ Jesus, who live [and] walk not after the dictates of the flesh, but after the dictates of the Spirit. For the law of the Spirit of life [which is] in Christ Jesus [the law of our new being] has freed me from the law of sin and of death.
Romans 8:1–2, AMPC

Today we will be dealing with accusations like judgment, condemnation, guilt and shame.

The Bible warns us in Matthew 7:1 not to judge, criticize or condemn others unfairly with an attitude of self-righteous superiority so that we too will not be judged unfairly because just as we judge others when we are sinful and unrepentant, so will we be judged with the same standard we used to pass out judgment. Inquire instead of judging others.

Also, in Matthew 7:3–5 Jesus asks us to examine ourselves before we point out the mistakes or wrongdoing of others. Why worry about a speck in your friend's eye, when you have a log in your own? How can you think of saying to your friend, 'Let me help you get rid of that speck in your eye,' when you can't see past the log in your own eye? So first get rid of the log in your own eye; then you will see well enough to deal with the speck in your friend's eye.

Living in the dark covers up sin but once we come in the light of Jesus, sin is revealed, so we can repent. Proverbs 28:13 says that He who conceals his transgressions will not prosper, but he who confesses and forsakes them will find compassion.

Conviction is the act of convincing a person of error or of compelling the admission of a truth. You have a conscience that lets you know right from wrong. If your conscience doesn't convict you then you know you keep God's commandments, so do the things that are pleasing in His sight and consistently seek to follow His plan for you (1 John 3:19–21). When we learn to practice the truth of God's Word, we come to the light. We come to right standing with God, and we have the desire to obey and live by His commandments (John 3:19–21).

The Bible says in John 16:8 that the Holy Spirit will convict the world of its sin, and of God's righteousness and judgment. The Holy Spirit brings correction when our spirit is receptive to Him, prompting us to repent of our sins and be restored to fellowship with God.

As children of God, we recognize His voice (John 10:5 & 27). Every child recognizes the voice of his father. When God speaks to us by His Spirit, we will know because it will be in alignment with His Word.

Galatians 6:1 gives us a guide to correct a person in sin. If anyone is caught in any sin and you are led by the guidance of the Holy Spirit. You are to restore the person in a spirit of gentleness, not with a sense of superiority or self-righteousness. A word of caution is given, keep a watchful eye on yourself, so that you are not tempted as well.

The story of the adulterous woman teaches us that before we point out others sin, we should make sure we are not guilty of sin (John 8:7). There's a saying that when you point one finger at someone the remaining four fingers are pointing back at you.

Constructive criticism? This seems like an oxymoron, a figure of speech with a contradictory term. It's just a way of giving positive and negative feedback in a friendly manner rather than an oppositional one and wrapping it up with encouragement. Constructive criticism is more likely to be accepted if the intent is focused on the improving recipient's work or behavior. For it to be effective, it should be delivered at a time when the person is ready and willing to receive it.

Has this ever happened to you? You find yourself criticizing someone for inappropriate behavior and before the week runs out, you are faced with similar temptations.

The Bible refers to the devil as the accuser of the brethren. That nagging voice that you hear constantly trying to convince you that you're no good and God will never forgive you. He wants to bring shame, guilt and condemnation on you, which are not from God. Romans 8:1–2 reminds us that we are not condemned if we live and walk by dictates of the Spirit, not the flesh. The enemy's aim is to make us feel guilt and shame to draw us further away from the Lord and deeper into sin. We must be alert and aware of his schemes. Resist the devil, and he will flee from you (James 4:7).

Get rid of all self-inflicted ideologies (thoughts). Ask loved ones, the people that you know genuinely care about you, to give you feedback on what they think about you. A way to let a compliment stick is to say thank you.

Take time to read through, understand and get familiar with the **Emotional Detox Process** on page 57. It will help you complete the steps below. Write down your "aha" moments, takeaways, answers and lessons in a journal so that you don't forget.

THE EMOTIONAL DETOX PROCESS

Reflect: Identify a past or current situation where you are experiencing accusations of judgment, condemnation, guilt and shame, and who is/was involved as it comes to memory.

How did you react to the accusations? When are you most vulnerable? Why did you feel condemned, guilty or ashamed? Prepare yourself.

Reveal: People's perceptions of others can reflect their own issues. Write down the answers revealed in your reflections. How did the experience(s) make you feel? Write down who was involved; you, others or an entity.

What part did you have to play? Did someone tell you they felt judged or condemned by what you did? Did you give in to self-pity, guilt or shame?

Release: Release the people or entities who have offended you based on how they made you feel, including yourself. Ask God what you can do to be healed. Ask for wisdom.

Say the prayer of faith below with a heart of repentance. Repeat it as many times as you need to do it to see change happen.

Dear God, wash me thoroughly from my iniquities and cleanse me from my sins by the blood of Jesus (mention any sins relating to judgment, condemnation, guilt and shame) **(Psalm 51:2).**

I confess my transgressions to you, LORD, forgive the guilt of my sin **(Psalm 32:5).**

I release the weight and burden of condemnation, guilt and shame. (Breathe in and out)

As I have freely admitted that I have sinned and confessed my sins, I believe that you are faithful and just and have forgiven my sins and cleansed me from all unrighteousness and everything not in conformity to Your will in purpose, thought and action **(1 John 1:9)** *in Jesus Name. Amen!*

Restore: Say the declarations below aloud to yourself with attention, power, strong desire, faith and persistence. Repeat it as many times as you need to until you see change happen.

- *I declare that I am born of God. I live by the dictates of the Spirit of God, not by my flesh. I am the righteousness of God in Christ Jesus. I have dominion over my sinful nature, therefore, I am not condemned.*

- *Jesus has set me free, so I am free from any judgment, condemnation, guilt and shame. I embrace holiness, living a consecrated life—a life set apart for God's purpose and in the fear of God.*

- *I am a new creature in Christ, the old things have passed away, everything is made new in Jesus Name. Amen!*

Response: If you are faced with a situation involving judgment, condemnation, guilt and shame, how will you respond? Read Matthew 18:15–17, AMPC below:

If your brother wrongs you, go and show him his fault, between you and him privately. If he listens to you, you have won back your brother. But if he does not listen, take along with you one or two others, so that every word may be confirmed and upheld by the testimony of two or three witnesses. If he pays no attention to them [refusing to listen and obey], tell it to the church; and if he refuses to listen even to the church, let him be to you as a pagan and a tax collector.

Day 8

<u>DEALING WITH DISCONTENTMENT</u>

*Not that I am implying that I was in any personal want, for I have
learned how to be content (satisfied to the point where I am not
disturbed or disquieted) in whatever state I am. I know how to be
abased and live humbly in straitened circumstances, and I know also
how to enjoy plenty and live in abundance. I have learned in any
and all circumstances the secret of facing every situation, whether
well-fed or going hungry, having a sufficiency and enough to spare
or going without and being in want.*
Philippians 4:11-12, AMPC

Today we will deal with discontentment; envy, jealousy, greed and lust.

In Philippians 4, Paul wrote to the people of God in Philippi expressing his gratitude for their concern towards him even though he had already discovered how to be content in whatever state he found himself in. He knew how to adjust to different life circumstances.

Discontentment arises when you are not satisfied with your current state of being or circumstance. You want more material possessions whether you can afford them or not. You are constantly looking at other people and comparing yourself and lifestyle with theirs. You want what other people have by any means possible. You let other people define the standard of living for you or your family. You're constantly looking around to make sure you keep up with them because they cannot out do you. You may even get a second job to keep up but that doesn't matter as long as you get what you want. All these lead to envy, jealousy, greed and lust.

There are a few times when people get discontented for a good reason. It may be time for a change for the better like an expansion. Time to try new things or opportunities in career, business or ministry. These individuals are not making changes because they compare their lives with other people.

With the advent of social media celebrities, people involved in such things make these "celebrities" their role models, and covert what they wear, and have, and do to emulate what they see on social media.

When you pay careful attention to your own work by examining your actions, attitudes and behaviors, then you can have the personal satisfaction and inner joy of doing something commendable without comparing yourself to another. Every person is responsible for their own faults, conducts and inadequacies (Galatians 6:4–5).

There is a distinction between jealousy and envy. To envy is to want something which belongs to another person. Exodus 20:17 says that *"You must not covet your neighbor's house. You must not covet your neighbor's wife, male or female servant, ox or donkey, or anything else that belongs to your neighbor."*

Envy wants what someone else has, but jealousy is when you're worried someone's trying to take what you have. If you want your neighbor's new luxury car, you feel envy. Envy is most often used to refer to a covetous feeling toward another person's attributes, possessions, or stature in life.

In contrast, *jealousy* is the fear that something which we possess (usually a special relationship) will be taken away by another person. Although jealousy can apply to our jobs, our possessions, or our reputations. Jealousy more often refers to anxiety which comes when we are afraid that the affections of a loved one might be lost to a rival.

We fear that our spouses, or perhaps our children, will be lured away by some other person who, when compared to us, seems to be more attractive, capable and successful.

Envy is a two-person situation, whereas jealousy is a three-person situation. Envy is a reaction to lacking something. Jealousy is a reaction to the threat of losing something (usually someone).

Greed is a selfish and excessive desire for more of something especially wealth, power or food. There is usually a very strong wish to continuously get more of these things.Another strong craving or desire, often of a sexual nature, is *lust*.

Most people focus on external factors instead of internal factors like how they look on the outside. There may be deeper issues on the inside that need to be addressed.

For example, a pastor received a gift of a new luxury car and some of the church members were offended thinking he bought it, so they started talking about it. After a few weeks, the pastor hands the keys to his luxury car to one of his congregation members who seemed to be offended by the car. The congregant received the keys with so much joy saying "Thank you!" Then the pastor asked him, "How come you can have it and I can't?" That right there is envy in the works, not offense.

The grass is always greener from the other side until you go there and find out that it isn't. We were all created to be unique with multiple talents. Find what you're good at. Don't try to be like someone else. You don't know what sacrifices they made to be where they are today. If you really had to wear their shoes, they probably would not fit. Find your identity in Christ. Not in the material things of this world, which are here today and gone tomorrow.

When you have a need, pray to God then He provides. Not long after that, another need will arise, so you present another request. Just make sure you stop to give thanks in between.

Take time to read through, understand and get familiar with the **Emotional Detox Process** on page 57. It will help you complete the steps below. Write down your "aha" moments, takeaways, answers and lessons in a journal so that you don't forget.

THE EMOTIONAL DETOX PROCESS

Reflect: Identify a past or current situation where you are experiencing discontentment like envy, jealousy, greed and lust. Note who is/was involved as it comes to memory.

List the reasons you feel discontent, how you react, and when you're most vulnerable, then prepare yourself.

Reveal: Write down the answers revealed in your reflections. Note how the experience(s) made you feel? Did you feel unworthy, unimportant, not good enough, unrecognized, unaccepted, etc.?

Who was involved: yourself, others or an entity like an organization, church, company, institution, etc.? What part did you have to play? Did you give in to envy, jealousy, greed or lust?

Release: Release the people or entities who have offended you based on how they made you feel, including yourself. Ask God what you can do to be healed. Ask for wisdom.

Say the prayer of faith below with a heart of repentance. Repeat it as many times as you need to until you see change happen.

> *Dear God, I come to You to ask for forgiveness for being jealous or envious of (insert name). Forgive me for my thoughts and actions because of envy, jealousy, greed and lust. Forgive me for not trusting in Your promise to supply all my needs. Wash me thoroughly and cleanse me from my sins by the blood of Jesus (mention any sins relating to envy, jealousy, greed and lust)* **(Psalm 51:2).**

> *I release the weight and burden of envy, jealousy, greed and lust, and how they made me feel (name the feelings you identified). (Breathe in and out.)*

> *I pray for the grace of God, your unmerited favor and blessing to reject and renounce all ungodliness and worldly desire. Give me the grace to live a discreet, moderate and self- controlled life. I grow in the knowledge of God and Jesus my Lord. And ask for more grace to live an upright and godly life in this present world* **(Titus 2:11–12)** *in Jesus Name. Amen!*

Restore: Say the declarations below aloud to yourself with attention, power, strong desire, faith and persistence. Repeat it as many times as you need to until you see change happen.

- *I declare that I am born of God. I live by the dictates of the Spirit of God, not by my flesh. I have dominion over my sinful nature, therefore, I am not envious, jealous, greedy or lustful of others.*

- *Jesus has set me free, so I declare that I am free from envy, jealousy, greed and lust. I set my mind on things that are above, not on earthly things (Colossians 3:2). By the Holy Spirit, I have self-control and develop patient endurance, godliness and brotherly affection with love for everyone (2 Peter 1:6–7).*

- *I am content in my present circumstances knowing that by His divine power, God gives me everything I need for life and godliness as I grow in the knowledge of Him (2 Peter 1:3). I seek first the Kingdom of God and His righteousness and He gives me everything I need (Matthew 6:33).*

- *I am content and self-sufficient through Christ, satisfied to the point where I am not disturbed or uneasy regardless of my circumstances. I know how to get along and live humbly in difficult times, and I also know how to enjoy plenty and live in abundance. I can do all things through Christ who strengthens and empowers me to fulfill His purpose. I am ready for anything and equal to anything through Him who infuses me with inner strength and confident peace (Philippians 4:11–13).*

Response: When you are faced with a situation involving discontentment, how will you respond?

Give thanks to God in all things and situations (1 Thessalonians 5:18). Express gratitude first. Give thanks for what you have no matter how little and watch God bless and multiply it. Giving thanks opens the door to receive more. Gratitude doesn't make you weak or make the person receiving it better than you.

You are uniquely you, don't try to be like someone else. If someone's life inspires you, let it inspire you to be a better version of yourself. No one has your fingerprint because God likes the uniqueness about you. If we both painted a picture, it wouldn't be exactly the same. We have different ways of expressing things. Even twins as much as they may look alike, have different personalities and ways of expressing themselves.

Celebrate and compliment others when they are successful. Don't try to steal their shine.

Surround yourself with people who genuinely love you. You can trust what your friend says, even when it hurts (Proverbs 27:6). Familiarity can cause people to downplay your success. It could also be a result of some insecurities they haven't addressed. Preserve your relationships by celebrating each other's uniqueness, strengths, gifts and talents.

Keep your life free from the love of money and be content with what you have, knowing that God will never leave you nor forsake you (Hebrews 13:5).

Day 9

DEALING WITH SELF- IDOLATRY

*For by the grace (unmerited favor of God) given to me I warn
everyone among you not to estimate and think of himself more highly t
han he ought [not to have an exaggerated opinion of his own importance],
but to rate his ability with sober judgment, each according to the degree
of faith apportioned by God to him. Live in harmony with one another;
do not be haughty (snobbish, high- minded, exclusive), but readily adjust
yourself to [people, things] and give yourselves to humble tasks. Never
overestimate yourself or be wise in your own conceits.*
Romans 12:3 & 16, AMPC

Today we will deal with self- idolatry; pride, arrogance, uncontrolled ego
and haughtiness.

Self- idolatry is when you shift the attention or focus that belongs to God
to yourself. You think more highly of yourself than necessary and have an
exaggerated opinion of your own importance.

At this point, you take the place of God in your life. It may not be intentional
but over time if you keep making yourself the object of attention, it becomes
self-idolatry. This in turn gives birth to pride, arrogance, uncontrolled ego
and haughtiness. This is why the very first commandment of The Ten
Commandments is *"You shall have no other gods before me"* (Exodus 20:3).

It is also why Jesus replied, *"Love the Lord your God with all your heart and
with all your soul and with all your mind,"* when asked *"What is the greatest
commandment?"* He said, *"This is the first and greatest commandment"*
(Matthew 22:37–38).

Pride is the feeling of satisfaction you get from your abilities or possessions.
You begin to trust your own abilities more than what God can do in your
life. You don't acknowledge Him for your success, recognizing that He is
the source of it all. When you put the focus on yourself and you remove
God from the picture, you open yourself up for an attack by the devil.
Arrogance is when people have an inflated opinion of their abilities

or possessions. Haughtiness is showing an attitude of superiority and believing that someone or something is unworthy of one's consideration or respect.

Ego is the idea or opinion that you have of yourself like the level of your ability and intelligence or your importance as a person. It is the part of us that needs to be special, seeks approval or feels lacking in some way. If it is not controlled, the ego can become very unhealthy.

Let's look deeper into pride. Pride is self-focused, thinks that he/she is better than others, rejects advice from others, rarely acknowledges flaws and often tends to blame others.

People work hard to achieve status, wealth and power. Pride wants other people to know how much they have achieved and what it takes to be like them without giving glory to God. They become so consumed with themselves in their thoughts that there is no room for God.

King Nebuchadnezzar of Babylon was a king God gave sovereignty, majesty, glory, and honor to. He made him so great that people of all races and nations and languages trembled before him in fear.

When his heart was lifted up and his spirit became so proud that he behaved arrogantly, he was deposed from his royal throne and his glory was taken away from him (Daniel 5:19–20).

Pride is not to be confused with confidence even though both qualities signify being able to use abilities, gifts and talents to accomplish a goal. Confidence focuses on using them to the fullest to bless others with good intentions and humility, while pride focuses on personal gain accompanied by arrogance and selfish intentions.

Confident people have a good understanding of their identity. They are aware of their strengths and weaknesses. They are open to criticism and advice from others to improve themselves and take responsibility for their actions.

There is a confidence that we have as children of God. It is total dependence on our God-given abilities while knowing that with God's strength, support and power, we can do all things.

Humility is an attitude or quality of mind [Acts 20:19] whereby a person holds a realistic view or opinion of his own goodness and importance. Humble people know when they sin or offend others and they don't hesitate to ask for forgiveness. They live in submission to God depending on Him to meet their needs. It is the opposite of pride, haughtiness, and self-exaltation.

Humility with the reverent fear of the Lord brings the reward of riches, honor, and life (Proverbs 22:4).

We must continually examine where our affections lie because we live in a culture that persistently promotes the idolization of people, things, and even self.

Take time to read through, understand and get familiar with the **Emotional Detox Process** on page 57. It will help you complete the steps below. Write down your ""aha"" moments, takeaways, answers and lessons in a journal so that you don't forget.

THE EMOTIONAL DETOX PROCESS

Reflect: Identify a past or current situation where you are experiencing self- idolatry: pride, arrogance, uncontrolled ego and haughtiness. Note who is or was involved as it comes to memory. What is the reason you feel proud, arrogant, egotistic, or haughty? When are you most vulnerable? Prepare yourself.

Reveal: Write down the answers revealed in your reflections. How did the experience(s) make you feel? Did you feel unworthy, unimportant, not good enough, unrecognized, unaccepted, empty, discontent, unhappy, etc.?

Who was involved; yourself, others or an entity like an organization, church, company, institution, etc.?

What part did you have to play? Did you give in to pride, arrogance, uncontrolled ego, haughtiness? Did you act snobbish, superior or pompous?

As you read through the following questions, be honest with yourself. If you answer yes to any of the following, there is a part of your soul that needs to be released from self- idolatry.

- Did you trust in your abilities, appearance, wealth and power more than you trust in God?

- Did you focus on outward appearance rather than what's in the heart of people involved?

- Did you always have to win? Were you more concerned about being right when making point?

- Did you gain satisfaction from other people's downfall when you had a personal gain or felt jealous when they did well?

- Did you compete for attention? Or did you end up making most things about you?

- Did you talk more about yourself in a conversation than you listened to others?

- Did you constantly compare yourself to other people who were better than or not as good as you?

- Did you talk about other people's flaws but wouldn't admit your own inadequacies?

Release: Release the people or entities who have offended you based on how they made you feel, including yourself. Ask God what you can do to be healed. Ask for wisdom.

Say the prayer of faith below with a heart of repentance. Repeat it as many times as you need to until you see change happen.

*Dear God, I come to you to ask for forgiveness for giving in to pride, arrogance, uncontrolled ego and haughtiness. Forgive me for my thoughts and actions as it relates to self-idolatry. Forgive me for trusting in my abilities, appearance, wealth and power more than I trust in you, God. Wash me thoroughly and cleanse me from my sins by the blood of Jesus (mention any sins relating to pride, arrogance, uncontrolled ego and haughtiness) **(Psalm 51:2)**.*

I release the weight and burden of pride, arrogance, uncontrolled ego, haughtiness. (Breathe in and out.)

*I pray for the grace of God to be humble and submit myself to God. **(James 4:6–7)**. And more grace to live an upright and godly life in this present world. **(Titus 2:11–12)** in Jesus Name. Amen!*

Restore: Say the declarations below aloud to yourself with attention, power, strong desire, faith and persistence. Repeat it as many times as you need to until you see change happen.

- *I declare that I am born of God. I live by the dictates of the Spirit of God, not by my flesh. I have dominion over my sinful nature, therefore, I do not yield to the desires of the flesh, the desires of the eyes and pride in possessions **(1 John 2:16)**.*

- *Jesus has set me free, so I declare that I am free from pride, arrogance, uncontrolled ego, and haughtiness. I set my mind on things that are above, not on earthly things **(Colossians 3:2)**.*

- *I am a love being. I love the Lord my God with all my heart, with all my soul and with all my mind **(Matthew 22:37)**.*

- *I seek first the Kingdom of God and His righteousness and acknowledge that He is the source of all my blessings **(Matthew 6:33)**.*

- *I do not brag or become proud or arrogant **(1 Corinthians 13:4)**. I make my boast in the Lord; whether I eat or drink, or whatever I do, I do all for the honor and glory of God **(1 Corinthians 10:31)**.*

- *I boast that I understand and know You, Lord; that You are Yahweh who desires and shows unfailing love, justice, and righteousness on the earth **(Jeremiah 9:24)**.*

- *By the power of the Holy Spirit, I walk in meekness, humility, gentleness, and lowliness of mind. I am not conformed to this world but transformed by the renewing of my mind **(Romans 12:2)**.*

- *I humble myself [feeling very insignificant] in the presence of the Lord, and He exalts me, lifts me up and makes my life significant **(James 4:10)** in Jesus Name. Amen!*

Response: If you are faced with a situation involving self-idolatry, how will you respond?

> *Look here, you who say, "Today or tomorrow we are going to a certain town and will stay there a year. We will do business there and make a profit." How do you know what your life will be like tomorrow? Your life is like the morning fog—it's here a little while, then it's gone. What you ought to say is, "If the Lord wants us to, we will live and do this or that." Otherwise, you are boasting about your own pretentious plans, and all such boasting is evil (wrong). Remember, it is sin to know what you ought to do and then not do it.* ***(James 4:13–17, NLT)***

Give thanks to God in all things and situations (1 Thessalonians 5:18). Express gratitude first. Give thanks for what you have no matter how little and watch God bless and multiply it. Gratitude doesn't make you weak or make the person receiving it better than you.

Celebrate and compliment others when they are successful. Don't try to steal their shine. Preserve your relationships by celebrating each other's uniqueness, strengths, gifts and talents.

Day 10

<u>DEALING WITH ADDICTIONS AND CRAVINGS</u>

He has made everything beautiful and appropriate in its time. He has also planted eternity [a sense of divine purpose] in the human heart [a mysterious longing which nothing under the sun can satisfy, except God]—yet man cannot find out (comprehend, grasp) what God has done (His overall plan) from the beginning to the end.
Ecclesiastes 3:11, AMP

Jesus replied to them, "I am the Bread of Life. The one who comes to Me will never be hungry, and the one who believes in Me [as Savior] will never be thirsty [for that one will be sustained spiritually].
John 6:35, AMP

Today we will deal with addictions and cravings. There is a God size void in every person that only God can fill. There are longings, hunger and thirsts in every human heart that only God can satisfy. When you become saved, your body becomes the temple of the living God, His Holy Spirit dwells in you (1 Corinthians 3:16).

You shouldn't allow other things to compete for room in your heart with God. Your heart was made to contain God, but when you have other desires or cravings, they gradually take the place of God in your life. This is the reason that the greatest commandment is *"Love the Lord your God with all your heart and with all your soul and with all your mind"* (Matthew 22:37).

God satisfies the thirsty and fills the hungry with good things (Psalm 107:9). Jesus declared in John 6:35 that He is the bread of life. Whoever comes to Him will never go hungry, and whoever believes in Him will never be thirsty again. Those who are hungry and thirsty for righteousness are blessed because they will be satisfied (Matthew 5:6).

Whoever drinks the water He gives will never thirst and this water becomes a spring of water, satisfying the thirst for God which continually flows and bubbles up into eternal life (John 4:14).

A *craving* is an irresistible and intense desire or longing for something.

It is also an unexplainable urge you get when you long for something or someone's attention. It arises to satisfy emotional needs, such as calming stress and reducing anxiety. The things we crave usually leave a good feeling and have many enjoyable memories associated with them.

Food cravings prompted by emotions are typically for foods containing fat, sugar, or both, which may lead to weight gain if you continually yield to the cravings. It takes either a mindset that you're not deprived of the unhealthy options or God empowering you to make healthy choices.

The progression of continued satisfaction of cravings is an addiction. When people are addicted to something, they are constantly thinking about it, worried about it, planning around it and eating it if it is edible.

The *cycle of addiction* begins by rewarding yourself with something to avoid a bad feeling or negative emotion. This creates a dependency because of the temporary relief or satisfaction you get when you have it. You are satisfied for a few moments then you want more of it. The repetition of this cycle creates an addiction.

During the 12 Day Power Detox Program, you may have experienced withdrawal symptoms (headaches, acne, loss of concentration and irritability) from different food items like coffee, sugar, fast food or processed food. These are signs of addiction.

A person could be addicted to a substance or an activity. Types of addiction range from everyday drugs like alcohol and cocaine to behaviors like gambling, stealing, eating, dieting, pornography, using the internet, playing video games, working, exercising, shopping, etc. These preoccupations take your attention from God and you begin to rely on the addiction when subjected to any kind of stress or emotional difficulty.

The Bible says in Philippians 2:13 that it is not in your own strength that you are able to overcome temptation, or whatever might offend God and discredit the name of Christ. It is God who is effectively at work in you to strengthen, energize and create in you the power, desire and the ability to fulfill your purpose for His good pleasure. When we are repetitively doing things to please God, it is not an addiction. Where there is an addiction issue, this is not the case. People can depend on addictions to satisfy emotional displeasure as they manage negative emotions like sadness, anxiety, anger, boredom, loneliness and frustration.

When a person allows addiction to overtake their actions, they can become distracted from the people in their lives and their responsibilities. They also become more interested in thinking and talking about the addiction than any other topic.

Addiction isn't just something you experience. It can take control over different areas of your life. No matter how terrible you behave and how horrific the sins you commit during addictive behaviors, you can rid yourself of that former way of the flesh and receive life by the Holy Spirit which gives you a new beginning.

When we give into either craving or addiction, it is important to recognize our own powerlessness and let God take care of us. With this faith in Him comes the strength to lead the lives we want, free of cravings and addictions.

Here are a few scriptures for meditation.

"No test or temptation that comes your way is beyond the course of what others have had to face. All you need to remember is that God will never let you down; he'll never let you be pushed past your limit; he'll always be there to help you come through it. So, my very dear friends, when you see people reducing God to something they can use or control, get out of their company as fast as you can" (1 Corinthians 10:13–14, MSG).

"So, let God work his will in you. Yell a loud no to the Devil and watch him scamper. Say a quiet yes to God and he'll be there in no time. Quit dabbling in sin. Purify your inner life. Quit playing the field. Hit bottom and cry your eyes out. The fun and games are over. Get serious, really serious. Get down on your knees before the Master; it's the only way you'll get on your feet" (James 4:7–10, MSG).

Blessed is the man who remains steadfast under trial, for when he has stood the test he will receive the crown of life, which God has promised to those who love him. Let no one say when he is tempted, "I am being tempted by God," for God cannot be tempted with evil, and he himself tempts no one. But each person is tempted when he is lured and enticed by his own desire. Then desire when it has conceived gives birth to sin, and sin when it is fully grown brings forth death. (James 1:12–15, ESV)

Take time to read through, understand and get familiar with the **Emotional Detox Process** on page 57. It will help you complete the steps below. Write down your "aha" moments, takeaways, answers and lessons in a journal so that you don't forget.

THE EMOTIONAL DETOX PROCESS

Reflect: Identify a past or current situation where you are experiencing addictions and cravings, and the types of addictions and cravings as it comes to memory.

When are you most vulnerable to addictions and cravings? Think about how it all started and what the triggers are. Prepare yourself.

Reveal: Write down the answers revealed in your reflections. Note how the experience(s) made you feel? Did you feel unworthy, unimportant, not good enough, unrecognized, unaccepted, empty, discontent, unhappy, etc.? Which feeling or negative emotion were you reacting to?

Who was involved; yourself, others or an entity like an organization, church, company, institution, etc.? What part did you have to play? Did you give in to your addictions and cravings?

What things have a greater priority than God in your life? What is your greatest addiction? The answer to that reveals who or what is number one in your life.

Try this little exercise: Make a list of all the things that are important to you. Anything about which you might say, "I don't know how I could live without this." Number the list in order of priority, one being most import-ant. You can make "God" all-encompassing (His Word, His church, His Son, His Spirit, worshiping Him, etc.). Examine the top three items. How does God rank?

Now let's examine food cravings. As you read through the following questions, be honest with yourself. If you answer yes to any of the following, there may be a part of your soul that needs to be released from addictions and cravings. It could also be a sign of nutritional deficiencies.

- Do you crave chocolate? It may not be getting enough magnesium in your diet.

- Can't get enough salt? You could be too stressed, and, in turn, harming your adrenal glands. Research shows that salt cravings are often due to a calcium deficiency.

- Do you crave sugar frequently? Sugar cravings often indicate that you have low or fluctuating blood sugar. You may not be eating a balanced diet or missing some essential nutrients in your diet. Healthy fats and protein provide slow and steady forms of energy. Other reasons such as lack of sleep, stress and hormone imbalances cause intense sugar cravings. Sugar gives you quick energy so when you don't eat enough calories, your body starts looking for fuel fast as a way to catch up.

Release: Release the people or entities who have offended you based on how they made you feel. Take responsibility for giving in to cravings and allowing addictions to take root in your heart and forgive yourself.

Ask God what you can do to be healed. Ask for wisdom.

Say the prayer of faith below with a heart of repentance. Repeat it as many times as you need to until you see change happen.

Dear God, I come to you to ask for forgiveness for giving in to addictions and cravings (name them). Forgive me for my thoughts and actions as it relates to addictions and cravings (forgive other people involved). Forgive me for trusting in addictions and cravings (name them) more than I trust in You, God.

Wash me thoroughly and cleanse me from my sins by the blood of Jesus (mention any sins relating to addictions and cravings) (Psalm 51:2). I release the weight and burden of addictions and cravings (name them and the emotions you felt). (Breathe in and out.)

I place my life before you God as an offering. I give You my sleeping, eating, going to work, and walking-around life. I depend on You God for my daily needs and I fix my attention on You because You are my source. I readily recognize what You desire of me, and quickly respond to it. Help me to be patient as You bring the best out of me, transforming and progressively changing me into what You created me to be **(Romans 12:1–2).**

By the grace of God, His unmerited favor and blessing, I reject and renounce all ungodliness, temptation and worldly desire to live discreet, moderate and self-controlled. I grow in the knowledge of God and Jesus my Lord. And I ask for more grace to live an upright and godly life in this present world **(Titus 2:11–12)** *in Jesus Name. Amen!*

Restore: Say the declarations below aloud to yourself with attention, power, strong desire, faith and persistence. Repeat it as many times as you need to until you see change happen.

- *I declare that I am born of God. I live by the dictates of the Spirit of God, not by my flesh. I have dominion over my sinful nature, therefore, I do not yield to the desires of the flesh, the desires of the eyes and pride in possessions* **(1 John 2:16).**

- *Jesus has set me free* **(John 8:36),** *so I declare that I am free from addictions and cravings (name them). He filled me with the spirit of power, love and a calm and well-balanced mind and discipline and self-control* **(2 Timothy 1:7).**

- *I am not conformed to this world but transformed by the renewing of my mind (Romans 12:2). I set my mind on things of the Spirit so I have life and peace* **(Romans 8:5–6).**

- *I am complete in Christ and I am self-sufficient in Christ's sufficiency.*

- *I am a love being. I love the Lord my God with all my heart, with all my soul and with all my mind* **(Matthew 22:37).**

- *I seek first the Kingdom of God and His righteousness and* acknowledge that He is the source of all my blessings *(Matthew 6:33)*.

- By the power of the Holy Spirit, I have self-control and develop patient endurance, godliness and brotherly affection with love for everyone *(2 Peter 1:6–7)*.

- I clothe myself with the presence of my Lord Jesus Christ and I make no provision for [nor even think about gratifying] the flesh or its desires *(Romans 13:13–14)*.

- I resist addictions, cravings and temptations (name them) through Christ who strengthens and empowers me in Jesus Name. Amen *(Philippians 4:13)*.

Response: If you are faced with a situation involving addictions and cravings, how will you respond?

"Everything is permissible for me, but not all things are beneficial. Everything is permissible for me, but I will not be enslaved by anything [and brought under its power, allowing it to control me]" **(1 Corinthians 6:12, AMP).**

"For we do not have a High Priest Who is unable to understand and sympathize and have a shared feeling with our weaknesses and infirmities and liability to the assaults of temptation, but One Who has been tempted in every respect as we are, yet without sinning. Let us then fearlessly and confidently and boldly draw near to the throne of grace (the throne of God's unmerited favor to us sinners), that we may receive mercy [for our failures] and find grace to help in good time for every need [appropriate help and well-timed help, coming just when we need it]" **(Hebrews 4:15–16, AMPC).**

Watch the company you keep. Paul's assertion is reasonable when he says in 1 Corinthians 15:33, *"Bad company ruins good morals."* When you hang around with someone who has the same addiction or craving problems, they will be a bad influence on your life.

"Watch and pray so that you will not fall into temptation. The spirit is willing, but the flesh is weak" **(Matthew 26:41, NIV)**.
"Call upon me in the day of trouble; I will deliver you, and you will hon-

or me" **(Psalm 50:15).**

Having respect for God and faith in Him is sometimes enough to get some-one through a craving. The answer isn't always to remove the addictions from our lives. The answer is to love God MORE! We must allow ourselves to be "filled with all the fullness of God."

Day 11

POWER OF SPOKEN WORDS

*Let no foul or polluting language, nor evil word nor unwholesome or worthless talk [ever] come out of your mouth, but only such [speech] as is good and beneficial to the spiritual progress of others, as is fitting to the need and the occasion, that it may be a blessing and give grace (God's favor) to those who hear it. And become useful and helpful and kind to one another, tenderhearted (compassionate, understanding, loving-hearted), forgiving one another [readily and freely], as God in Christ forgave you. **Ephesians 4:29 & 32, AMPC***

Death and life are in the power of the tongue, And those who love it and indulge it will eat its fruit and bear the consequences of their words.
Proverbs 18:21, AMP

Today we will discuss the power of the spoken word and deal with sin associated with the spoken word like gossip, lying, exaggeration, slander, backbiting and swearing.

Words are powerful. They can build up or break down, encourage or destroy. The words you release out of your mouth can either create a good thing or a bad thing.

Words have no geographical limitation. Jesus sent His word and the centurion's servant was healed in the same hour (Matthew 8:13).

Your words also have the power to create life or death because as Jesus is so are you in this world (1 John 4:17). Your words shape your life so be careful what you say to yourself and others.

"Your words are continually educating others around you. They reveal your focus, confidence, expectations and what is comfortable to you."
– Dr. Mike Murdock

Ephesians 4:29 tells us to avoid *"any unwholesome talk."* The verse goes on to say that our speech should be good and helpful for building up and encouraging others according to their needs. Our words should also benefit them as they listen. So, there are two steps you need to take concurrently. First, do not use bad language. Second, use words that will bless and give grace to those listening. Use words that are pure, kind and encouraging.

By your words, you will be justified and acquitted, and by your words, you will be condemned and sentenced (Matthew 12:37). Words are seeds (Luke 8:5–15). Over time they are planted, watered and they produce the type of fruit in which the words were conceived (Luke 6:44). Positive words produce positive results, while negative words produce negative outcomes.

Luke 6:45 says a good man brings good things out of the good stored up in his heart and an evil man brings evil things out of the evil stored up in his heart. The mouth speaks what the heart is full of.

Your mind works like a tape recorder. Everything you say or hear other people say is recorded and can be played back to you at any point in time. So, if you form a habit of saying positive things, positive thoughts will be recorded and you will think positively and do the right things. The chain connecting heart and tongue cannot be broken. For good or bad, it will always be there. Try this, before you speak, pause and ask yourself, "What am I about to say? What is my motive?"

The Bible says in James 3:8–10 that no one can tame the human tongue; *it is a restless evil [undisciplined, unstable], full of deadly poison. With it we bless our Lord and Father, and with it we curse men, who have been made in the likeness of God. Out of the same mouth come both blessing and curs-ing. These things should not be this way [for we have a moral obligation to speak in a manner that reflects our fear of God and profound respect for His precepts].* This verse doesn't give a solution to this problem.

James 1:26 also says that if you claim to be religious but don't control your tongue, you are fooling yourself, and your religion is worthless. When the tongue is not controlled, people fall into sin by gossiping, lying, exaggerat-ing, slandering, backbiting and swearing.

To control what comes out of your mouth, you have to monitor what goes into your mind and watch what you meditate on. The gates into your mind and heart are your eyes and ears. Be careful what you listen to and feed your eyes with. Fix your mind on what is true, honorable, right, pure, fair, appropriate [decent], lovely, kind, pleasant, gracious and admirable. Think about things that are excellent and worthy of praise (Philippians 4:8).

Gossip is idle talk or rumor about the personal or private affairs of others, typically involving details that are not confirmed as being true. The result of gossip is always broken trust and hurt feelings even if the people talking didn't mean direct harm. God's Word warns us to stay away from people who gossip and to guard our words when we speak about others.

Your motive determines whether news becomes gossip. If your intentions are good, you can bring the gossip to a grinding halt and turn it into something positive. But if you just want to pass on the latest piece of juicy information, then it's gossip.

Slander is the next progression to gossip. *Slander* is described as gossip with evil intent for the sole purpose of ripping apart someone's reputation. The Bible also refers to slander defining it as making a false statement that damages a person's reputation. Slander can destroy someone's marriage, job, wealth, and family.

Backbiting is hateful talk about someone who is not present. It's like gossip but more malicious and with more evil intent. Backbiting, gossip, lies and slander often lead to division, strife, and suspicion. These are Satan's strategies to destroy reputations and break up relationships. The Bible warns us in 2 Timothy 2:16 to avoid all empty talk that is irrelevant, vain, useless, worthless, ungodly and idle. Because it will lead people into more and more ungodliness.

Exaggeration is a statement that implies something is larger, more important, better or worse than it really is.

Lying is simply not saying the truth. It is also disguising the truth by not saying the real facts or communicating accurate information. The Bible says in Proverbs 12:22 that lying lips are extremely disgusting to the Lord but those who deal faithfully are His delight. If we know lying is wrong, why do we do it? Here are a few reasons. We fear the consequences of telling the truth (See Genesis 18:10–15). Lying can be more convenient than telling the truth. Lying can make us look good to our friends like saying, "Yeah, I got an A on the test, too." No reason can justify a lie. Telling the truth is always the best option. Yes, you might get grounded. And true, you may not look as good in front of your friends. But those are short-term consequences. Our long-term integrity is at stake every time we choose between telling a lie and telling the truth. "Truthful lips endure forever, but a lying tongue lasts only a moment" (Proverbs 12:19).

Swearing includes several types of inappropriate language like cursing, profanities and obscenities. If you are prone to swearing, you should look up the meaning of the words you say. It is a real eye-opener!

> *But above all, my fellow believers, do not swear, either by heaven or by earth or with any other oath; but let your yes be [a truthful] yes, and your no be [a truthful] no, so that you may not fall under judgment (James 5:12, AMP).*

A *curse* is said to "wish for evil or misfortune to befall someone." Here's what the Bible says, "Bless those who persecute you; bless and do not curse" (Romans 12:14). Nobody said it would be easy, but you can give it a try. When someone hurts us, we want to hurt back. But God obviously says that's wrong. 1 Peter 3:9 says, "Do not repay evil with evil or insult with insult. On the contrary, repay evil with blessing, because to this you were called so that you may inherit a blessing."

Profanity is socially offensive language which is indecent and disrespectful speech or action, even against something sacred such as the name of God. This breaks God's heart in a big way. That's why it's one of the Ten Commandments: *"You shall not misuse the name of the Lord your God" (Exodus 20:7).*

Obscenities are morally repulsive and disgusting and include all other forms of foul language, often sexual in nature. Dirty jokes fall into this category. Again, the Bible is clear: "Nor should there be any obscenity, foolish talk or coarse joking, which are out of place" (Ephesians 5:4). Also, "Rid yourself of ... filthy language" (Colossians 3:8).

Take time to read through, understand and get familiar with the **Emotional Detox Process** on page 57. It will help you complete the steps below. Write down your "aha" moments, takeaways, answers and lessons in a journal so that you don't forget.

THE EMOTIONAL DETOX PROCESS

Reflect: Identify a past or current situation where you are experiencing gossip, lying, exaggeration, slander, backbiting and swearing. Who was involved as it comes to memory? How do you react? When are you most vulnerable to the ill spoken words? What was the reason you engaged in gossip, lying, exaggeration, slander, backbiting and swearing? Prepare yourself.

Reveal: Write down how the experience made you feel? Did you feel insecure, unwelcomed, rejected, betrayed, unimportant, desperate, not good enough, etc.? Who was involved? Are you angry towards God, yourself, others or an entity?

What does your word say about you? Do you keep blaming others for your emotions without owning up to your own mistakes? What part did you have to play? Did someone tell you they were offended by what you said?

Does putting down another person make you feel better? Do you feel secure in God's love? What is the enemy's trying to steal from you? Unity, joy, peace, love, etc.

Release: Release the people or entities who have offended you based on how they made you feel, including yourself. Ask God what you can do to be healed. Ask for wisdom.

Say the prayer of faith below with a heart of repentance. Repeat it as many times as you need to until you see change happen.

Dear God, I come to You to ask for forgiveness for giving in to gossip, lying, exaggeration, slander, backbiting and swearing. Forgive me for my thoughts and actions as it relates to ill-spoken words from my tongue (forgive other people involved if you were the recipient). Forgive me for blessing and cursing from the same mouth I praise You with. Wash me thoroughly and cleanse me from my sins by the blood of Jesus (Psalm 51:2).

I release the weight and burden of gossip, lying, exaggeration, slander, backbiting and swearing. (Breathe in and out.)

Set a guard, O Lord, over my mouth; Keep watch over the door of my lips to keep me from speaking thoughtlessly **(Psalm 141:3).**

I readily recognize what You desire of me, and quickly respond to it. Help me to be patient as You bring the best out of me, transforming and progressively changing me into what You created me to be **(Romans 12:1–2).**

By the grace of God, I refuse to gossip, harm or speak evil of others with my words, I will keep my words and promises even when it hurts **(Psalm15:3)**. *I love my enemies, bless those who curse me; do good to those who hate me; pray for those who speak evil about me; mistreat me; accuse me falsely and persecute me* **(Matthew 5:44)**. *I receive more grace to live an upright and godly life in this present world* **(Titus 2:11–12)** *in Jesus Name. Amen!*

Restore: Say the declarations below aloud to yourself with attention, power, strong desire, faith and persistence. Repeat it as many times as you need to until you see change happen.

- *I declare that I am born of God. I live by the dictates of the Spirit of God, not by my flesh. I have dominion over my sinful nature, therefore, I do not yield to the desires of the flesh. I live blamelessly and do what is right God's sight, speaking the truth from a sincere heart.*

- *Jesus has set me free (John 8:36), so I declare that I am free from gossip, lying, exaggeration, slander, backbiting and swearing. He filled me with the spirit of love, power and a calm and well-balanced mind and discipline and self-control (2 Timothy 1:7).*

- *I am not conformed to this world but transformed by the renewing of my mind (Romans 12:2). I set my mind on things of the Spirit, so I have life and peace (Romans 8:5–6).*

- *I meditate and fix my mind on the truth, things that are worthy of reverence, honorable and appropriate [decent], things that are just, pure, lovely and lovable, kind, pleasant and gracious. I fill my mind with things that have virtue, excellence and is worthy of praise (Philippians 4:8).*

- *I am a love being, so I love others as I love myself.*

- *By the power of the Holy Spirit, I have self-control and develop patient endurance, godliness and brotherly affection with love for everyone (2 Peter 1:6–7).*

- *I clothe myself with the presence of my Lord Jesus Christ and I make no provision for [nor even think about gratifying] the flesh or its desires (Romans 13:13–14).*

- *I resist the temptations to gossip, lie, exaggerate, slander, backbite and swear through Christ who strengthens and empowers me in Jesus Name. Amen! (Philippians 4:13).*

- *I speak only words that are good and helpful for building up and encouraging others and benefit them as they listen (Ephesians 4:29).*

- *I strive to live in peace with everybody and pursue that consecration and holiness (Hebrews 12:14).*

Response: If you experience a situation with gossip, lying, exaggeration, slander, backbiting and swearing, how will you respond?

How you respond or react to it will determine if you have been totally healed from past experience.

When you feel upset about a wrong done against you, write out your complaints in a journal explaining to God how you feel about certain people or incidents. By telling them to Him, you don't need to tell others.

When you communicate, always start with giving thanks before you look at the negative outlook on life or your current unpleasant situation. Start with one thing you are thankful for during the experience, and then state your displeasure in the most loving way possible so that your conversation will be gracious, pleasant and attractive. When you do this, you will have the right response for everyone (Colossians 4:6).

Love people genuinely and surround yourself with people who do the same. When you have a genuine love for the others according to 1 Corinthians 13:4–7, it simply isn't possible to speak evil of them.

You can trust what your friend says, even when it hurts (Proverbs 27:6). Preserve your relationships by speaking good things about others.

When you hear a rumor or story about someone, don't tell it to someone else. Let it end with you. "Fire goes out without wood, and quarrels disappear when gossip stops" (Proverbs 26:20).

Meditate on God's Word and pray. Fill your mind with the Word of God so that your speech will reflect it and you will have it as a guide against a temptation to fall into sin. When you sin, ask God for forgiveness and for His help to keep your speech clean and pure (1 John 1:9).

Day 12

<u>DEALING WITH REJECTION</u>

For the sake of his great name the Lord will not reject his people, because the Lord was pleased to make you his own. ***1 Samuel 12:22, NIV***

Be strong and courageous. Do not be afraid or terrified because of them, for the Lord your God goes with you; he will never leave you nor forsake you." ***Deuteronomy 31:6, NIV***

What, then, shall we say in response to these things? If God is for us, who can be against us? ***Romans 8:31, NIV***

Today we will deal with rejection and abandonment.

Rejection is the act of not accepting, believing, or considering something or someone. God created us to be loved, accepted and appreciated. People can feel rejected when they are not accepted as good enough for a purpose. Rejection can be experienced when someone is not allowed to join a group, organization, or institution. Denial of privilege can also cause feelings of rejection.

Rejection happens to everyone. Rejection can happen on the job, in relationships, groups we belong to or anywhere else. We may not have control over when it happens to us, but we can control how we respond to it.

If you've experienced rejection you are not alone, Jesus experienced rejection too (John 15:18). He was rejected by His peers, half-brothers, nation, the Gentiles and the world He created (John 1:10).

In the hour of His agony, He was betrayed by one friend, denied by another, and abandoned by the majority of His disciples. He experienced loneliness, suffering, grief, and rejection. He was despised and rejected by mankind, a man of suffering Who was familiar with pain (Isaiah 53:3). He did this to bear our griefs, sicknesses, weaknesses and distresses. To carry our sorrows and pains on the cross of Calvary (Isaiah 53:4).

Rejection can destroy our self-esteem, and attacks who we are and our purpose in life. This is why it is one of the most common tools the devil will use to destroy a person's life. God never wanted us to feel rejected or abandoned. He desires for you to know who you really are, and realize how deeply God loves, accepts and appreciates you, so that you can live out the fullness of all God has ordained you to be.

"Rejection is a divine announcement that you have finished a relationship and God is going to move you into a new realm. An obstacle is a divine announcement that God is getting ready to maximize hidden potential"
– Dr. Cindy Trimm.

The Bible says that we are fearfully and wonderfully made, and we are created in the image and likeness of God (Psalm 139:14; Genesis 1:27). There is greatness on the inside of you because God lives in you (1 John 4:4) and you need to know that. Discover God's purpose for your life and create your identity in what God's Word says about you. Base your value and self-worth on what God's Word says.

Rejection may simply mean they are not the right person God wants to use to help you. There's someone else you need to meet. Trust Him to send the right person. Sometimes it takes experiencing rejection before we realize that it is time to move on or be separated from a relationship. It shows that they don't have room for your greatness. It's possible that they are intimidated by your presence and what you bring to the table.

Are you ready to experience rejection or obstacles knowing that God is about to shift and change some areas and relationships in your life?

Abandonment means to withdraw one's support or help from, especially despite duty, allegiance or responsibility. It also means to desert or abandon a friend in trouble. A person may feel abandoned due to a parent's abuse or neglect or loss due to death, divorce and illness. Seeking a parent's approval is a sign that you're basing your identity on what they think of you. Don't get me wrong, parental approval is a good thing, but you may not always get it. Psalm 27:10 says *"Even if my father and mother abandon me, the LORD will take care of me."* Do you trust God to always be there for you?

When people experience rejection and abandonment, they start building impenetrable walls around them which makes it difficult to establish new relationships. It will eventually lead to loneliness which indicates the absence of a relationship with God, purpose and misplaced identity.

God promises to never to leave or forsake us (Hebrews 13:5 and Deuteronomy 31:8), so when our identity is based on what He says about us, we can be assured that we're not going to face rejection from Him.

Even after Jesus left this world, God gave us His Spirit to live within us (1 Corinthians 6:19). We are God's temple (1 Corinthians 3:16). We always have company, so we should not feel alone if we develop a relationship with the Holy Spirit. We can speak to Him and He speaks back to us.

Take time to read through, understand and get familiar with the Emotional Detox Process on page 57. It will help you complete the steps below. Write down your "aha" moments, takeaways, answers and lessons in a journal so that you don't forget.

THE EMOTIONAL DETOX PROCESS

Reflect: Identify a past or current situation where you are experiencing rejection and abandonment. Who was involved as it comes to memory? What area of your life it is affecting: marriage, career, health, business, etc.? How did you react to rejection and abandonment? When are you most vulnerable? Why did you feel rejected and abandoned? Prepare yourself.

Reveal: How did the experience make you feel? Did you feel unaccepted, irrelevant, unloved, insecure, angry, confused, sad, unwelcomed, lonely, betrayed, self-pity, hopeless, envy, jealousy, hate unimportant, desperate, not good enough, etc.? Who was involved? Are you angry with yourself, others, an entity or God? Do you blame Him for creating you a certain way?

As you read through the following questions, be honest with yourself. If you answer yes to any of the following, there is a part of your soul that needs to be released from rejection and abandonment.

- Do you keep blaming others for your emotions without owning up to your own mistakes?

- Do you have a hard time admitting that you are wrong, or receiving constructive criticism? You may be basing your identity upon their ability to be right about everything.

- Do you blame yourself even before you know you are at fault? Do you question your self-worth?

- Did someone tell you they felt rejected or abandoned by your action?

- Did you experience rejection or abandonment in a past relationship that you have not healed from?

- Are you allowing your past experience to prevent you from building new relationships?

- Are you constantly afraid of being rejected, abandoned or being lonely?

- Do you feel the need to fit in or be accepted by others and be a part of everything?

- Do you feel secure in God's love and accepted by Him?

- Is your identity based on what your parents, mentors, friends or others think of you?

- What is the enemy trying to steal from you; identity, unity, joy, peace, love, etc.?

Release: Release the people or entities who have offended you based on how they made you feel, including yourself.

It is important that you process the pain felt by rejection especially in a close or intimate relationship so that you don't make negative decisions based on how you feel. The level of pain involved in rejection depends on the value you give to that relationship.

The goal of the enemy is to get us filled up on the inside with emotional baggage and negative feelings in our hearts against one another, ourselves, and God.

Ask God what you can do to be healed. Ask for wisdom. Say the prayer of faith below with a heart of repentance. Repeat it as many times as you need to until you see change happen.

> *Dear God, I come to You to ask for forgiveness for giving in rejection and abandonment. Forgive me for my thoughts and actions as it relates rejection and abandonment (name them). Forgive me for not trusting and believing in Your unfailing love and acceptance towards me. (Forgive other people involved if you were the recipient.) I ask that You forgive me for holding it against them this long. I receive the complete healing of my soul. Wash me thoroughly and cleanse me from my sins by the blood of Jesus (Psalm 51:2).*
>
> *I release the weight and burden of rejection and abandonment. (Breathe in and out.) Lord, help me to no longer be agitated, disturbed, fearful, intimidated and unsettled about the situations I face in life (John 14:27).*
>
> *Free me from the spirit of timidity (of cowardice, of craven and cringing and fawning fear), and fill me with the spirit of power, love and a calm and well-balanced mind and discipline and self-control (2 Timothy 1:7).*
>
> *Help me to be patient as You bring the best out of me, transforming and progressively changing me into what You created me to be (Timothy 12:1–2).*
>
> *I pray the God, Who gives hope, will bless me with complete happiness, joy and peace because of my faith. And may the power of the Holy Spirit fill me with hope (Romans 15:13) in Jesus Name. Amen!*

Restore: Say the declarations below to reaffirm your identity in Christ. Repeat it as many times as you need to until you see change happen.

- *I declare that I am born of God (1John 5:18). I have received the Spirit of God (1 Corinthians 2:12). He dwells within me, so I am not alone.*

- *I am a child of God (John 1:12). Even if my father and mother abandon me, the LORD will take care of me. He will not forget me (Isaiah 49:15).*

- *I am part of God's chosen people, the royal priesthood and holy nation, a people belonging to God (1 Peter 2:9, 10).*

- *I am partaker of God's divine nature (1 Peter 1:4).*

- *I am seated with Christ in the heavenly realm (Ephesians 2:6).*

- *I am a friend of Jesus. He revealed to me everything that He has learned from the Father (John 15:15).*

- *I am Christ's ambassador (2 Corinthians 5:20). I represent Him and represent Him to the world.*

- *I am complete in Christ. I have the fullness of life filled with the Father, Son and Holy Spirit (Colossians 2:10).*

- *Jesus has set me free (John 8:36), so I declare that I am free from the weight and burden of rejection and abandonment. I am free from condemnation (Romans 8:1). He filled me with the spirit of power, love and a calm and well-balanced mind and discipline and self-control (2 Timothy 1:7).*

- *God loves me dearly. Nothing can separate me from the love of God (Romans 8:35).*

- *Because I am precious in God's eyes, honored, and He loves me, He gives men in return for me, peoples in exchange for my life (Isaiah 43:4).*

- *I have been blessed with every spiritual blessing (Ephesians 1:3). I am a love being, so I love others as I love myself.*

- *I declare that God's grace and power are enough for me when I feel rejected or abandoned. He promises to never leave me or forsake me.*

- *By the power of the Holy Spirit, I have self-control and develop patient endurance, godliness and brotherly affection with love for everyone (2 Peter 1:6–7).*

- *Because the Lord strengthens, helps and upholds me with His righteous right hand, my life is free from fear and anxiety (Isaiah 41:10).*

- *God has a plan for me, plans for welfare and not for evil, to give me a future and a hope (Jeremiah 29:11).*

- *I strive to live in peace with everybody and pursue that consecration and holiness (Hebrews 12:14) in Jesus Name. Amen!*

Response: If you experience a situation with rejection and abandonment, how will you respond? How you respond or react to it will determine if you have been totally healed from past experience.

Meditate on God's Word and pray. Fill your mind with the Word of God so that your actions will reflect it and you will have it as a guide against the temptation to fall into sin. When you sin, ask God for forgiveness and His help to keep your speech clean and pure (1 John 1:9).

Make bold declarations based on God's Word. Speak the words continuously until they produce the desired result in you and others. Your words shape your life. A good rule of thumb is to repeat the declarations for at least five minutes, three times each day; morning, mid-day and evening. You can also do it as many times you want in a single day. The more you hear them, the quicker they will transform your thinking.

It's ok to grieve about a relationship for a while. Grieving is a natural part of the human experience but don't let it turn into depression or an excuse to withdraw your involvement from people and life. Meet with good friends, eat healthy meals, exercise, do the activities you enjoy and stay present with your feelings.

CHAPTER 6

SUCCESS STORIES & TESTIMONIALS

SUCCESS STORIES

I had an amazing experience during the 12 Day Power Detox Program. I never thought I could do it until I actually started. It was really helpful in forming healthy habits and I felt good emotionally and spiritually at the end. I also lost 15 pounds. It's been a year now and I have only gained 5 pounds back since the program.

– Pastor Roseline O. Whitby, ON Canada
12 Day Power Detox Ambassador

The 12 Day Power Detox Program is a healthy way to lose weight and improve emotional well-being. It was challenging at the beginning but the snacks, especially the nuts, were really helpful in keeping up my energy.

The results were awesome. Not only did I lose weight, but I also stopped eating unhealthy foods and started eating healthy foods and snacks. I experienced improved bowel movement, skin texture, sleep at night and I felt energized all day long.

It's hard to pick a favorite but these smoothies are the ones I liked the most: Tropical Paradise, Heavenly Green Joy, Triple Berry Love and Berry Delight Smoothies.

I recommend this program to any one physically and emotionally drained, you will definitely regain your strength and be emotionally fit. I felt good reading the devotionals daily and connected with the Word of God.

Thanks, Ade, for sharing it with us. I will be sharing my experience with friends and family and doing the detox again.

What I like most about the Detox Program is that it is designed to benefit the whole you—spirit, soul and body. Weight loss is just an added benefit. I lost a little over 12 pounds and 2 inches off my bust, waist and hips. I am now a converted "smoothie lover" and I have incorporated these smoothie recipes into my diet, especially for breakfast.

– Dr. Modele O., Atlanta, Georgia
12 Day Power Detox Ambassador

This 12 Day Power Detox Program is a great way to jumpstart your fitness lifestyle and rejuvenate your spirit, soul, and body.

When Ade told me about this program, my initial reaction, as a physician was "I don't do detox." I also did not like smoothies. But Ade, in her gentle and persuasive manner, said to me, "Why don't you give it a try?" So, I decided to sign up for the program.

I browsed through the e–book and went grocery shopping with my 6-year-old daughter. This was a great opportunity to teach her about making healthy choices while grocery shopping and show her how to do it.

I must say the initial few days were not easy on my body. I had headaches, which I later discovered were due to inadequate intake of water. This is addressed in the "Frequently Asked Questions" section of this book. The "easy to follow" and "no fitness equipment required" exercise videos provided in the Private Facebook Support Group were also very helpful. I looked forward to receiving the devotions every day.

By the third day, my body had fully adjusted to the routine and I began to see the benefits of the Detox Program.

Even my co-workers noticed the difference and said to me "Dr. O, you look so fresh and beautiful this morning, what's going on?" I shared this program with them and some of them signed up.

The Holy Banana Smoothie and the Tropical Paradise Smoothie are some of my favorites. For someone, who did not like smoothies, the quantity was just right, and the taste was perfect. When I felt hungry during the day, I had one serving of the recommended healthy snacks between the smoothie meals. My daughter was a great supporter, counting down the days with me. She enjoyed helping me make the smoothies, measuring and blending the ingredients and even tasted the smoothies on occasion.

What I like most about the Detox Program is that it is designed to benefit the whole you—spirit, soul and body. Weight loss is just an added benefit. I lost a little over 12 pounds and 2 inches off my bust, waist and hips.

My advice to first-timers to the Detox Program is to read the book thoroughly. It has all the answers to your questions, especially the

"Frequently Asked Questions" and the "Important Notes" sections. Read the devotional daily, participate in the accompanying exercise video, and most of all, have fun!

I am now a converted "smoothie lover" and I have incorporated these smoothie recipes into my diet, especially for breakfast. As a cardiologist, I usually counsel my patients on adopting a healthy lifestyle that includes exercise and at least five servings of fruits and vegetables daily. The smoothies make it much easier to do this.

Finally, I want to encourage you to join us on this exciting fitness journey as we maintain a healthy spirit, soul and body in 2019!

By Day 11, I had lost 8 pounds. My belly fat had melted off and my clothes fit better. I felt clean on the inside. Overall, I felt lighter, my skin looked fresher, and I had more energy, better bowel movement and rest at night.

– Dr. Tomi A., Chicago, Illinois
12 Day Power Detox Ambassador

I found out about the 12 Day Power Detox at the time when I was ready to get rid of the weight I gained during my last pregnancy.

Ade told me about her new program and she assured me that even though it is not a weight loss program, it would help me get started on my weight loss journey. After I received and read the e- book for the Program, I knew it was what I needed to do. I went grocery shopping the next day to buy everything I needed. Purchasing is made extremely easy with clear instructions.

I started on a Monday morning. I woke up early to blend my smoothies and packed my snacks so I was ready for Day 1. As I noticed the results each day, I was encouraged to continue the detox. By Day 11, I had lost 8 pounds. My belly fat had melted off and my clothes fit better. I felt clean on the inside.

Overall, I felt lighter, my skin looked fresher and healthier, I had more energy, and even bowel movements changed for the better. I saw myself substituting meals with some of my favorite smoothies even after the Detox Program. My favorite smoothies are the Tropical Paradise, Heavenly Green Joy and Apple Serenity Smoothie.

It's been a month since I completed the 12 Day Power Detox Program and I've been able to keep the 8 pounds off. I am more conscious about what I put in my body. I have continued refraining from drinking soda which was nearly a daily habit.

As a medical doctor, I personally and professionally recommend the Detox Program for anyone looking to jumpstart a healthier lifestyle. I have been sharing this great news with my friends and family.

———————————————————

The first thing I noticed after Day 2 was more regularity in my bowel movements. My body felt a lot lighter and I started sleeping longer hours at night. After Day 7, I checked my weight and I was down 4 pounds. I became more energetic. Even though this is not a weight loss program, I lost a total of 7 pounds and 3 inches off my waist.

– Grandma Jo, Houston, Texas
12 Day Power Detox Ambassador

I was excited to find out about the 12 Day Power Detox because it was an answered prayer.

I started the Program on Monday, October 30, 2017, and completed it on Friday, November 10, 2017.

The first thing I noticed after Day 2 was more regularity in my bowel movements. My body felt a lot lighter and I started sleeping longer hours at night. After Day 7, I checked my weight and I was down

4 pounds. I became more energetic. Even though this is not a weight loss program, I lost a total of 7 pounds and 3 inches off my waist.

I also noticed my skin was more radiant. The other day I went to see my new doctor for a routine medical checkup and the first thing she said was that I am looking younger than my age and whatever I am doing to keep this youthful look, I should continue.

My favorite smoothies are the Heavenly Green Joy Smoothie and the Triple Berry Love Smoothie. I love the taste of the smoothies and their effects on my bowel movements. Drinking the recommended amount of water daily also helped in many ways.

The 12 Day Power Detox Program was a very pleasant experience for me and I highly recommend everyone to experience the great benefits from it. I will be doing it again in the near future. I must add that it takes a lot of determination to get the positive results from the Program. I wish everyone a successful completion.

I lost 8 pounds in 11 days and during those days I noticed that my face and skin were smoother. I felt light after the program. This Program reset my whole system. I definitely recommend doing the Program.

– Ms. TJ A. Houston, Texas
12 Day Power Detox Ambassador

I've always known about the Program but was hesitant about doing this. I didn't think I could survive on fruits and vegetables for 11 days. I decided to try it out because I had been at a particular weight for a while and wasn't losing despite all attempts.

The first few days were hard, but I kept at it and got the desired results. I lost 8 pounds in eleven days and I felt light after the Program. During those days, I noticed that my face and skin were smoother plus I felt energized all day long.

I underestimated the effectiveness of the Salt Water Cleanse. If you try this, expect frequent bowel movements and make enough time for the cleansing process if you are doing it on a work day.

My favorite smoothies were the Tropical Paradise, Holy Bananas, Triple Berry Love and Berry Delight Smoothies. Pecans were my favorite snack choice.

After completing the Program, I realized eating fruits and veggies are very easy when I make them into smoothies and my water drinking habit improved.

I will be doing the detox again. I'm so glad I gave it a try.

I am more mindful about food overall and am proud to have lost 8 pounds in all! I lost 3 inches in my waist. The devotional helped me focus on the intent of my participation and were often right on time for the things I was facing during the detox.

– Ms. LaSetta H., Glendale, Arizona
12 Day Power Detox Ambassador

My participation in the 12 Day Power Detox Program definitely made a big impact on my lifestyle. I am more mindful about food overall and am proud to have lost 8 pounds in all! I lost 3 inches in my waist, 1 inch on my hips, and almost an inch in my bust area.

I tried the Salt Water Cleanse, it wasn't bad. It worked very well. I'm more aware of my intake and desire for sweets. I am working hard to make smarter choices.

My favorite smoothies are the Holy Bananas Smoothie, Triple Berry Love Smoothie and Apple Serenity Smoothie. I plan to continue having a smoothie at least once per day for a meal.

My favorite snacks were popcorn, avocado, and the detox tea.

I would recommend this Program to anyone that desires to make a change in their physical health and spiritual well-being. The devotional helped me focus on the intent of my participation and were often right on time for the things I was facing during the detox.

I will be doing the detox again in the near future.

I lost 6 pounds during the Detox Program. I gave my digestive system a break. I feel so rejuvenated, more alert in the morning; my skin was clearer, and I felt inner peace and unusual strength each day.

– Pastor Abimbola L., Colonia, New Jersey
12 Day Power Detox Ambassador

The Program is so valuable, it's not just for your body but also for your soul and spirit as Ade shares devotions to encourage you daily while living just on smoothies and some healthy nuts.

I lost 6 pounds during the Detox Program. I gave my digestive system a break. I feel so rejuvenated, more alert in the morning; my skin was clearer, and I felt inner peace and unusual strength each day.

Your Week 1 groceries may cost you $60–$70 if you shop at Whole Foods but it's worth it because you don't need any extra spending (Starbucks, lunch, etc.) for the rest of the week.

On Day 4, I could not believe how much energy I had, just depending on Green Smoothies. I felt very light and refreshed. Almonds were my favorite snacks and my favorite smoothie is the Holy Bananas Smoothie. I snack healthier now. I eat carrots and almonds instead of candy and chocolate bars. I rarely eat sweet pastries like bagels, donuts, or cake since I ended my detox.

It was a reminder to do many things I know, especially the power of my thoughts and words. It challenged me to think and speak more positively.

This is something to share with friends and loved ones. I shared the Detox Program with ladies at my church after I started it, and a few of them embarked on the journey and have great testimonies.
Ade has done an excellent job laying out the meal plan. She also provided the grocery list and where to shop. I plan to do it quarterly. I encourage everyone to go for it now and do it with a friend, spouse or sibling. Do not procrastinate.

the grocery shopping together and planned the meals (smoothie and salad) together. It was a refreshing experience for both of us. It brought us closer as we were experiencing the same results and we were always discussing our energy levels, dealing with hunger and the results we were experiencing like an improved bowel movement and sleep at night.

Tropical Paradise Smoothie and Heavenly Green Joy Smoothie were my favorites. I also made my own recipes based on the availability of fruits and vegetables I had. The mixed nuts helped me to curb hunger pangs. I drank the recommended amount of water as well as the detox teas. I was able to stop unhealthy eating and sugar cravings. Now I have smoothies every morning and I have removed starchy foods from my diet.

The Program kept me focused on the things that were important; work, family, etc. I realized I was in touch with myself; mind, body and spirit. In addition, I lost 7 pounds by Day 12 and 2 inches off my waist. Thanks for recommending this Program, we'll both do this again.

I LOVE this Detox Program!!! The focus is not just about the physical well-being but the spiritual, emotional and mental well-being. I lost 2 pounds by the morning of Day 3 and 5 pounds total by Day 10. The smoothies are delicious, and I enjoyed all of them. It was a good way to model to my kids healthier eating habits since I always challenge them to make healthier choices. I now avoid foods with added sugars and eat more raw greens.

– Ms. Michele S, Atlanta, GA

I started off great! Loved the smoothie from Day 1. I lost 2 pounds by the morning of Day 3, and 5 pounds total by Day 10. The fast became more challenging on Day 6. Probably because I was making several meals for the family in preparation for the week. I also started Daniel Fast earlier in the month so that could have contributed to the challenge so I modified from there on.

I LOVE this Detox Program!!! The focus is not just about the physical well-being but the spiritual, emotional and mental well-being. The smoothies are delicious, and I enjoyed all of them. It was a good way to model to my kids healthier eating habits since I always challenge them to make

---

I had amazing energy by Day 3. I didn't need coffee to be awake or maintain stamina. I began to lose weight immediately. I actually lost a total of 12 pounds. and everyone around me was astonished! My skin was clear, and makeup went on very smoothly.

– Ms. Shawn J., Maplewood, New Jersey

I am usually not quite a fan of "detox." I generally believed it was a glorified diet. However, after beginning, the first two days were the most difficult. I wondered, even with my prior minimal eating and living on coffee, could I really be addicted to sugars, salts, and other processed items? I quickly found my answer as I experienced severe headaches and nausea! However, as my body adjusted to this new style of eating it began to comply.

I had amazing energy by Day 3. I didn't need coffee to be awake or maintain stamina. I began to lose weight immediately. I actually lost a total of 12 pounds and everyone around me was astonished! My skin was clear, and makeup went on very smoothly.

I think the most positive point here is the weight stayed off! I also embraced the idea of eating healthy and thinking about food choices. Finally, I realized I could maintain this style of living, with less food, healthier food choices, and helping others make better choices.

Daily devotions also reminded me that detoxing is just as much about the soul as it is the body! When we feel good on the inside, we have a profound effect on our outside world, including our temple— the human body and the world at large!

I lost a total of 10 pounds. My skin glowed and my body experienced a lot of transformation (inches- wise) in my clothes. I was able to wear some clothes that I had sown and couldn't fit into before the detox.

– Pastor Favor W., Durham, North Carolina

It was tough though just feeding on smoothies. I felt tired initially but as time went on, things got better. I had cravings, but I drank my smoothie instead of snacking.

I lost a total of 10 pounds. My skin glowed and my body experienced a lot of transformation (inches-wise) in my clothes. I was able to wear some clothes that I had sown and couldn't fit into before the detox.

Making my smoothie without any dairy was awesome. That was a good discovery. My favorite smoothies are the Tropical Paradise Smoothie, Holy Bananas Smoothie, and Triple Berry Love Smoothie.

I did the Salt Water Cleanse. Wow! I will say it was effective. There was an improvement in my bowel movement.

I had more energy and felt energized all day long. Overall, I will do it again soon.

I lost 8 pounds. I went from 196 to 188 pounds in the 12 days and I still weigh 188 pounds almost a month later. The devotional helped me focus on the spiritual side of this journey and increased the joy of the Lord in me.

– Pastor Kouami A., Glendale, Arizona
12 Day Power Detox Ambassador

I didn't think that it was going to be that easy for me since it was the first time I was going to feed myself on smoothies alone. The awesome thing was I enjoyed most of the smoothies.

I lost 8 pounds. I went from 196 to 188 pounds in the 12 days and I still weigh 188 pounds almost a month later. My target weight is 175 and I hope to get there through this Program.
Tropical Paradise Smoothie, Holy Bananas Smoothie, Apple Serenity Smoothie, and Berry Delight Smoothie were my favorites. My favorite snacks to eat during the detox were cashew nuts and raw almonds.

I felt energized all day long during the 12 Day Power Detox Program.

The devotional helped me focus on the spiritual side of this journey and increased the joy of the Lord in me.

I was able to control my eating habits and stop craving unhealthy foods. I now eat smaller portions of foods and I'm still enjoying the smoothies. My bowel movement also improved.

I will be recommending the 12 Day Power Detox Program to my family and friends, and I will be doing it again soon.

I lost 10 pounds, developed new healthy eating habits and had more energy and better mood. I was more aware of what I eat, and I was able to curb my cravings for rice. The devotional helped me mentally know that God is always with me in anything I do.

– Ms. Kabeth D., St. Louis, Missouri

I lost 10 pounds, developed new healthy eating habits and had more energy and better mood. I was more aware of what I eat, and I was able to curb my cravings for rice.

The devotional helped me mentally know that God is always with me in anything I do.

My favorite smoothies are the Tropical Paradise Smoothie and Berry Delight Smoothie. I drank the recommended detox teas, 64 ounces of water daily and exercised more than three hours a week just on the smoothie diet.
Overall, it was a great experience mentally, spiritually and physically. This experience taught me that I can do all things through Christ. It also taught me how to help my body quickly adapt to any situation.

I will be recommending the 12 Day Power Detox Program to my family and friends. Thank you for allowing me to be part of this experience, it was a blessing and I will be doing the detox again.

I felt full of energy to do my daily tasks. I also lost 10 pounds and felt lighter. It killed my cravings for carbs and sugar, and I found that I loved eating vegetables again.

– Ms. Osen I., Chicago, IL

I incorporated the detox with the Daniel Fast, the first two weeks I only drank smoothies and then the latter part was with salads and very few cooked meals.

I was able to stop my cravings for sugar and eating carbs, and developed new healthy eating habits like more vegetables in my diet and more smoothies. I had more energy every day.

My bowel movement and skin appearance also improved. I felt full of energy to do my daily tasks. I also lost 10 pounds and felt lighter. It killed my cravings for carbs and sugar, and I found that I loved eating vegetables again.

Heavenly Green Joy Smoothie is my favorite smoothie. I drank the recommended detox teas and 64 ounces of water daily.

I will be recommending the 12 Day Power Detox Program to my family and friends, and I will be doing it again soon.

The Program was the reset button I needed for my diet and fitness. I lost about 7 pounds. My mind is clearer, and my clothes fit better. I was able to stop eating late at night and I now have better-eating habits. I enjoyed the devotion on forgiveness the most. It changed me so much. I reached out to someone who hurt me so deeply many years ago for reconciliation.

– Pastor Mayowa I., Chicago, IL
12 Day Power Detox Ambassador

The Program was the reset button I needed for my diet and fitness. I lost about 7 pounds. My mind is clearer, and my clothes fit better. I was able to stop eating late at night and I now have better-eating habits.

I enjoyed the smoothies very much. My favorite smoothie is Apple Serenity Smoothie. The ingredients combined very well. I did not feel hungry very much and when I did the nuts, carrots and popcorn helped. I felt energized all day long and I exercised for more than three hours a week during the detox.

The devotions made it easier because I could keep my mind on God and His Word instead of what my body was feeling. It helped to make this more than a physical struggle. The spiritual aspect made it easier to get through it.

I enjoyed the devotion on forgiveness the most. It changed me so much. I reached out to someone who hurt me so deeply many years ago for reconciliation. I first forgave them after reading the devotion and then reached out to them. For some reason, I had never consciously forgiven them. It really ministered to me that day and I was able to do so.

I did the Salt Water Cleanse on the Day 2 and it was so effective. It was easy to drink and gentle on the stomach. I'll continue with the smoothies, using them to replace at least one meal a day.

Thank you, Ade, for putting it together. I am now back to exercising regularly and I feel so good about it.

The program was a refreshing experience for my husband and I as we discussed the results, we experienced during the Detox Program, which were the same. I was able to stop unhealthy eating and sugar cravings. Now I have smoothies every morning and I have removed starchy foods from my diet. The Program kept me focused on the things that were important; work, family etc. I realized I was in touch with myself; mind, body and spirit. In addition, I lost 7 pounds by Day 12 and 2 inches off my waist.

– Ms. Nneka O., Brampton, ON, Canada

My husband and I did the 12 Day Power Detox Program together. We did healthier choices. I now avoid foods with added sugars and eat more raw greens.

The devotions were tremendous in helping with my emotional well-being. Staying focused and spending time in God's Word was my favorite part of the program.

God's Word is life and health to my whole body (Proverbs 4:22). Personally, the emotional weight loss and the spiritual gain from the Detox Program outweighs the physical weight loss. This is true "weight loss" that'll withstand time and I believe will eventually manifest outwardly in the physical body.

I had a few ""aha" moments but I'll just address the first two. One of the scriptures in the Day 3 Devotion, Matthew 18:35, "...forgive FROM YOUR HEART..." I don't think I had previously paid attention to the "your heart" phrase.

Another realization was that I was letting my experiences harden my heart. I had been saying for a few months now that I had lost my tears. Now I realize it was from a hardening heart, which has possibly affected my interactions with others and strangers.

I did struggle with getting 64 ounces of water with a limited solid intake. I think this also led to an infrequent bowel movement.

The bath soak was soothing and refreshing! I am looking forward to doing this detox again and to starting and finishing strong next time.

I didn't think I would be able to complete it but I'm glad I did. I lost a total of 10 pounds. I noticed my skin felt smoother. I also experienced better bowel movements. I have become more conscious of what goes into my mouth.

– Pastor Temitope A., Chicago, Illinois

I didn't think I would be able to complete it but I'm glad I did. I lost a total of 10 pounds. I noticed my skin felt smoother. I also experienced better bowel movements. I have become more conscious of what goes into my mouth. I like snacking but I have now adopted healthier snacks like peppers, carrots and nuts. I enjoyed trying different nuts. I also liked the chia seeds. And, I really enjoyed the Holy Bananas Smoothie.

I loved the effect of the Salt Water Cleanse on my bowels. The first time I did it was more effective than the second time.

The days I read the devotional, I was conscious about letting go of unforgiveness and putting God first place as my desire.

I plan on doing the detox again in the future.

TESTIMONIALS

First of all, I absolutely love each and every concept about the Detox. I have to be honest and share that I didn't do the very best at preparing on Friday but, this is now something I'm planning on doing quarterly. I would love to share it with my loved ones, due to the impact it's made in my soul, spirit and body.

I lost 7 pounds which is fair and I'm a lot more conscious about what I'm going to allow in my life as a whole. Thank you so much Ade for being a blessing to my life. You are a true daughter of our King
and an inspiration to so many.

Ms. Kamille M.

I usually do a Daniel Fast in January. This year, I joined your Detox Program which in many ways is quite similar. I did not follow the recipes strictly.

I've lost 8 pounds! I'm still on the Daniel Fast so still counting. I'm more alert and eating healthier than ever. Thank you for sharing your Program!

Ms. Tochi O.

The first day I was extremely hungry, so I added some chia seeds in my shake and found that helped. The first week went well but I think the timing is off for me to do this cleanse. It was really cold here; about 15 degrees and I found myself craving warmer foods. The cold smoothies made me shiver. The second week I only did morning and lunch smoothies and ate with my family at night. I continued to have a smoothie in the morning, tried the plant protein for the first time and liked it.

I loved the devotions. They were awesome, and I am a firm believer in healing in the body, soul and spirit. I am so proud of your accomplishment and hope for great success in the future.

Ms. Debbie H.

SHARE YOUR SUCCESS STORIES!

Nothing makes us happier than to hear how we make you happy!

Did you complete the 12 Day Power Detox with awesome results?

Please share your observations, challenges,
results and positive feedback by completing the
survey at *www.itstimefitnessaz.com/12dpd-survey*

or Email us at *info@itstimefitnessaz.com*

BECOME A 12 DAY POWER DETOX AMBASSADOR

You can become a 12 Day Power Detox (12DPD) Ambassador by completing the Detox Program, sharing your results and success story with us and the people you know will benefit from this Program. Your success story will be featured on our website or in our newsletter. To complete the survey, please visit *www.itstimefitnessaz.com/12dpd-survey*

ABOUT THE AUTHOR

ADE ASHAYE | HOLISTIC HEALTH COACH | FITNESS INSTRUCTOR

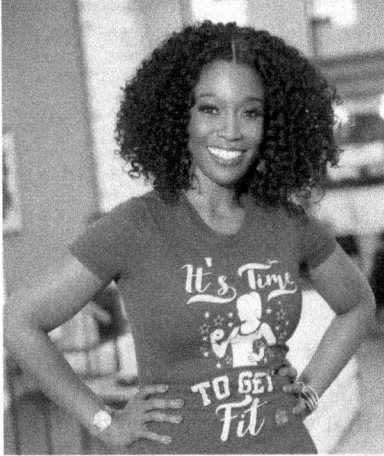

Ade, as she is popularly known, is the CEO of It's Time Fitness. She is a Holistic Health Coach who has helped people around the world experience transformation; spirit, soul and body.

She is a certified Fitness Nutrition Specialist, a motivational speaker and a sought-after Dance to Fitness™ instructor. She has appeared on several TV and radio shows as well as being featured in conferences and events in Canada and the United States.

With the release of her Fitness DVD, Dance to Fitness™ Party, her reach has extended to other parts of the world in Africa, Europe and Australia. Through her Fitness for Africa Initiative, It's Time Fitness is also making an impact in Africa, motivating people to get fit and spread the good news of health and wellness.

She was born and raised in Nigeria, moved to Canada to complete her undergraduate degree in civil engineering and now lives in the United States, pursuing her career, passion and purpose.

As a trained emotional healing minister, she has over six years of experience helping people around the world, not only to lose weight and be physically fit but also to release emotional baggage. She has offered nutrition and spiritual guidance to many people who are now living testimonies of the transformation they experienced as a result of working with her. Her passion comes from her personal experience with weight loss, love for the holistic lifestyle and her relationship with Jesus.

OTHER PROGRAMS OFFERED BY IT'S TIME FITNESS

DANCE TO FITNESS WORKOUT DVD

Dance to Fitness™ is a dance fitness program combining different group activities with a variety of fitness formats to Christian music from around the world to create a workout that will really move you—spirit, soul and body—in a positive and supportive atmosphere.

The workout features Scriptural declarations to engage the mind and spirit; fast, moderate and slow tempo music combined with cardio and strength training to tone and sculpt your body while burning fat. Dance to Fitness™ is for everyone, regardless of your age or size. Participants burn up to 800 calories per hour while having fun, losing weight and getting fit.

Host a Dance to Fitness™ Party in your city. The Dance to Fitness™ Party is an event full of fun and fitness activities that will help you get the tools you need to embrace a healthy and fit lifestyle.

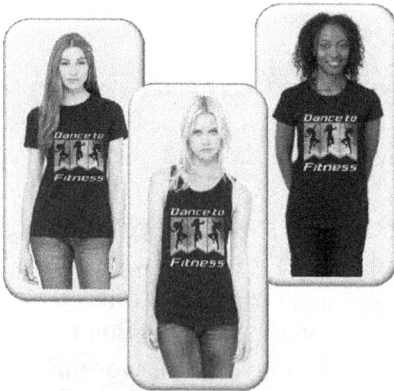

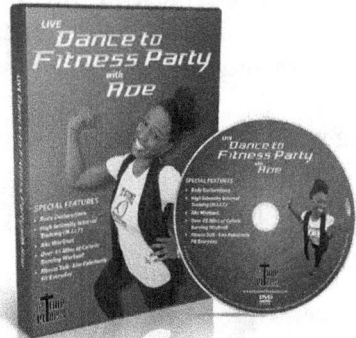

**AVAILABLE AT
WWW.ITSTIMEFITNESSAZ.COM**
Hurry while supplies last.....

The Dance to Fitness™ Party has been featured at various events and conferences around North America and Africa. Partner with us to bring the Dance to Fitness™ Party to your city and put your city on the fitness map!

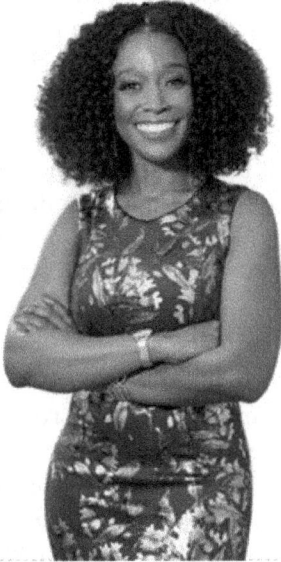

ARE WE A FIT? *Complimentary* **DISCOVERY** *Session*

⇒ *Uncover what is unconsciously sabotaging you from losing weight.*
⇒ *Discover how you can start losing weight now and begin to look fit and fabulous.*
⇒ *Recover your inner beauty and confidence with proven weight loss strategies to look good and feel good.*

LET'S FIND OUT »

COMPLIMENTARY 30 MINUTE DISCOVERY SESSION

This is a complimentary 30-minute scheduled phone call to help you:

- Uncover what is unconsciously sabotaging you from losing weight.

- Discover how you can start losing weight now and begin to look fit and fabulous.

- Recover your inner beauty and confidence with proven weight loss strategies to look and feel good.

FABULOUSLY FIT – 8 WEEK FITNESS & WEIGHT LOSS PROGRAM

The Fabulously Fit Program is an intensive 8-week Fitness and Weight Loss Program which was created by Divine inspiration, JUST FOR YOU! It will help you begin your journey to achieving and maintaining a healthy weight through dietary changes which lead to a lifestyle that includes healthy eating, regular physical activity, and balancing your calorie intake.

The goal is not to drastically change your diet but to take small steps that will eventually accumulate and translate into the big changes you desire. The unwanted weight will come off too, but it will be through a life-changing process.

The Fabulously Fit Program offers the following benefits:

1. The nutrition approach is a step-by-step process that will revolutionize your lifestyle and transform your body. It includes weekly life-changing nutrition exercises to help you achieve your nutrition goals, emotional well-being goals and your overall weight loss goals. Each week you will receive new recipes for delicious meals which will challenge you to form new healthy habits that will speed up your weight loss and get you in shape. You will also receive expert advice from a fitness nutrition specialist to create an effective nutrition and fitness plan that works for you and your family.
2. Prep Week: You get an additional week of support and guidance to help you prepare for the journey at hand. This includes a 30-minute introductory call with Ade.
3. Web-based Seminars covering in detail the areas that are unconsciously preventing you from losing weight and how you can overcome them to get lasting results. Included in Webinar Modules are assignments and worksheets to help you get a deeper and clearer understanding. Topics that will be covered, include: how to eat to lose or maintain weight; identify healthy food choices; serving size; money saving ideas for eating healthy; smart grocery shopping; reading nutrition facts label; breaking self-sabotaging eating and lifestyle habits; mindset shift to make a healthy lifestyle change; emotional eating; how to incorporate exercise into your lifestyle to maximize your results.

4. Three Group Coaching calls and one 30-minute private strategy call with Ade. The calls are to make sure you are progressing, to discuss your challenges and celebrate your victories. They will provide the added support and guidance you need during the challenge to stay focused on your health and fitness goals. Each session will be recorded and you will receive a MP3 file to refer to time and time again.

5. Learn how spiritual fitness is an important component of your physical fitness thru fasting and a devotional guide. You will also receive customized Bible scriptures for meditation that relate to your area of struggles. You will receive the audio version of It's Time Fitness - Body Declarations. The "Body Declarations" are powerful and spirit-filled confessions that have the power to transform your spirit, soul and body.

For more information about our programs and to contact us, please visit our website at **www.itstimefitnessaz.com**.

www.ingramcontent.com/pod-product-compliance
Lightning Source LLC
Chambersburg PA
CBHW050221270326
41914CB00003BA/511